UNDRUGGED: SLEEP

From Insomnia to Un-somnia -- Why Sleeping Pills Don't Improve Sleep and the Drug-Free Solutions That Will

Dr. Lori Arnold, PharmD

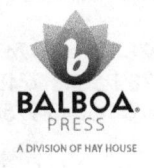

BALBOA PRESS
A DIVISION OF HAY HOUSE

Copyright © 2018 Dr. Lori Arnold, PharmD.

All rights reserved. No part of this book may be used or reproduced by any means, graphic, electronic, or mechanical, including photocopying, recording, taping or by any information storage retrieval system without the written permission of the author except in the case of brief quotations embodied in critical articles and reviews.

Balboa Press books may be ordered through booksellers or by contacting:

Balboa Press
A Division of Hay House
1663 Liberty Drive
Bloomington, IN 47403
www.balboapress.com
1 (877) 407-4847

Because of the dynamic nature of the Internet, any web addresses or links contained in this book may have changed since publication and may no longer be valid. The views expressed in this work are solely those of the author and do not necessarily reflect the views of the publisher, and the publisher hereby disclaims any responsibility for them.

The author of this book does not dispense medical advice or prescribe the use of any technique as a form of treatment for physical, emotional, or medical problems without the advice of a physician, either directly or indirectly. The intent of the author is only to offer information of a general nature to help you in your quest for emotional and spiritual well-being. In the event you use any of the information in this book for yourself, which is your constitutional right, the author and the publisher assume no responsibility for your actions.

Any people depicted in stock imagery provided by Thinkstock are models, and such images are being used for illustrative purposes only. Certain stock imagery © Thinkstock.

Print information available on the last page.

ISBN: 978-1-5043-9747-6 (sc)
ISBN: 978-1-5043-9748-3 (hc)
ISBN: 978-1-5043-9756-8 (e)

Library of Congress Control Number: 2018901550

Balboa Press rev. date: 03/22/2018

Contents

Introduction ix

Section 1 Are Sleep Drugs Worsening Your Insomnia?
Chapter 1   Insomnia: A Medical Indication in Need of a Drug ... 3
Chapter 2   Sleepless in America 7
Chapter 3   Trouble Sleeping? We Have a Drug for That 12
Chapter 4   The Truth About Z-Drugs: A Pharmacist's Synopsis ... 17
Chapter 5   Side Effects and Complications: Is the
            Benefit Worth the Risk? 30
Chapter 6   Complex Sleep-Related Disorders,
            Parasomnias, and "Zolpidem Zombies" 37
Chapter 7   Lawsuits and Legal Woes: The "Zolpidem Defense" 47
Chapter 8   Unvitamin Effect: Nutrient Depletions 49

**Section 2 From Insomnia to Un-somnia: Undrugged
            Solutions to Naturally Promote Sleep**
Chapter 9   The Undrugged Method 53
Chapter 10 Readjust: Adopt Better Sleep Habits 63
Chapter 11 Drug-Induced Disease: Drugs, Herbs,
            and Supplements That Can Cause Insomnia 78
Chapter 12 Replenish and Restore: Drug Alternatives 83
Chapter 13 Refresh: Healing with Food 100

Conclusion 117
Endnotes 119
Index 139

I alone cannot change the world, but I can cast a stone across the waters to create many ripples.

—Mother Teresa

Introduction
Becoming *Undrugged*: My Personal Mission

I used to be a human petri dish—a guinea pig for the pharmaceutical industry. Like many Americans, I bought into the philosophy that, if the government approved it and if my doctor prescribed it, my drug must be safe, right? I was wrong. Especially considering that every drug taken is designed to elicit a biological response, and chemicals notoriously don't just remain within the targeted organ or tissue. Keep adding more drugs to the mix, and inside your body, they will agitate and culminate into a festering toxic cocktail. Eventually this will become an accumulation of unintended consequences, or as I like to say, a party gone bad. Drugs do not always behave as intended, and more often than not they behave very badly.

Returning to my initial statement, notice I said in past tense, I *used* to be a human petri dish. I no longer adhere to the modern medical philosophy of "take a pill to cure the ill." I beat the malfunctioning medical system and found a solution that ultimately led to my self-healing. Embarking on my own personal wellness journey sparked the birth of the *undrugged* concept and created in me a desire to spread the word so others, like you, can benefit from my knowledge. You may be curious why a pharmacist, a drug expert and professional who dispenses thousands of prescription medications, would question the chemical marvels of modern medicine that pharmaceutical companies are endlessly producing. It is said, "Curiosity killed the cat." And I am a very curious person. On a daily basis, I started noticing patients were being placed on more and more drug therapies, and unfortunately, they were not getting better. In fact, the disturbing trend of overdrugging patients only contributed to declining health for many. Even as a pharmacist, I was not immune and experienced overdrugging firsthand; the experience helped me personally relate to the many disheartening stories of medical mishaps and subsequent drug-induced, long-term bodily damage.

Like many Americans, I was exposed to an onslaught of pharmaceutical drugs starting at a very young age. My parents were confused, stressed out, and fearful; therefore, they entrusted my well-being to my physician. Most parents, like my own, place considerable faith in the medical system, trusting each new diagnosis and ultimately adhering to all recommended treatment plans—after all, doctors are medical "experts." In my situation, with every new prescription written, my pediatrician hoped he was providing a cure I desperately needed to quell or eradicate my symptoms. As is the case with many sickly young children, the treatments quickly piled up.

At the age of six, I was diagnosed with asthma and allergies. Shortness of breath quickly morphed into severe bronchial restriction, chest tightening, labored wheezing, and excessive coughing. Medication was a necessity for my condition, but it came with consequences. Drug stimulation from theophylline and prednisone caused body twitching and shaking; sleep loss from intense night sweats and terrifying nightmares; bloodshot eyes with dark, puffy circles; and a red, irritated, and swollen face, to name a few of the physical manifestations and uncomfortable side effects resulting from drug therapy. Like a credit card ad, "Don't leave home without it," my albuterol inhaler was my safety blanket I kept in a nerdy fanny pack along with my spacer and peak-flow meter. I was completely dependent on, or more accurately *addicted* to, my "rescue" inhaler. I suffered multiple yearly hospitalizations from frequent viral and bacterial sinus and lung infections and was treated with countless steroid bursts, some lasting longer than thirty days, along with endless antibiotic courses.

With each passing year, drug after drug was prescribed for every new symptom I experienced. The snowball effect continued into my teens, with irregular menstruation and severe cystic acne, which led to treatment with oral contraceptives and more antibiotics. College stress and being a self-proclaimed overachiever landed me, once more, in the doctor's office for antidepressant medications and a series of antacids to treat my "sour" stomach. At twenty-four, I was diagnosed with cholecystitis, which led to the surgical removal of my gallbladder. Shortly thereafter, I was placed on continuous proton-pump inhibitor treatment with Nexium (esomeprazole) for worsening acid reflux and digestion issues. Chemically sustaining an environment of stomach acid suppression for eight years resulted in constipation and vitamin deficiencies; this meant adding more over-the-counter treatments—stool softeners; laxatives; and a myriad of supplements to correct low energy, dry skin, and hair loss. As you may suspect, I eventually developed insomnia and soon became dependent on Ambien (zolpidem) for sleep. By the time I was in my thirties, I took twelve prescription medications on a daily basis.

As I've demonstrated from firsthand experience, in the long-term, drugs often do not fix the problem, but instead contribute to deteriorating health and accelerated aging. Drugs often are Band-Aids used to quell symptoms, but rarely do they cure the ailment. With an average of seventy side effects per drug, every pill you take potentially burdens your health with undesirable or serious conditions, such as impaired gut function, weight gain, type 2 diabetes, hair loss, reduced thyroid status, hormone dysfunction, brain fog, increased potential for dementia, chronic constipation, and brittle bones. Many of these conditions become permanent, plaguing you for the rest of your life. Is this a risk you are willing to take?

Like myself, and millions of other Americans, you likely share the experience of taking a new drug only to find yourself bombarded by new symptoms completely unrelated to the original problem, which then led to another newly diagnosed disease, followed by more prescriptions. Drugs are commonly prescribed to "fix" the side effects of the first drug. Using myself as an example again, if you take Nexium (esomeprazole) for acid reflux for extended periods of time, you can subsequently develop constipation, acne, depression, and a vitamin B12 deficiency. This means you will now take Nexium, laxatives, and stool softeners, Accutane, Zoloft (sertraline) and Abilify (aripiprazole), along with B12 injections. Unfortunately, every added new drug introduces interactions and a tangle of more unintended symptoms, side effects, and even new diseases, justifying additional drug treatment. This overdrugging cycle happens every day in the modern American healthcare system. Overdrugging creates a type of codependent relationship with medications, causing you to rely heavily on synthetic drug effects to establish a sense of normalcy. Drugs become a safety blanket, providing a false sense of security and perceived health. Word to the wise, codependent drug relationships have no future—it's time to free yourself and break up with your drugs.

Why Should You Trust My Opinion?

I provided you a brief glimpse into my rapidly developing health crisis that prompted me to search for more viable answers and possible curative measures to preserve my body's wellness. A shift also had to occur in my professional life. I needed to step back and analyze my chosen career path and assess whether I was answering my soul's true calling; was I following my purpose in life? This introspective journey forced me to assess every career phase I've embarked upon and the choices that carved my professional story.

I have observed that a common complaint and source of contention for many consumers is, why should I trust your opinion? What are your credentials? If my doctor doesn't agree with alternative approaches, and he or she is the medical expert, why would I risk taking advice outside his or her recommendations? As I often say, even the most educated health care professionals "don't know what they don't know." There is a wealth of evidence-based literature and research supporting alternative medicine, which is ripe for the picking if one is inclined to devote time and energy to learning about it. Unfortunately, as it is not taught in medical school or pharmacy school, many practitioners quickly pooh-pooh this approach. I taught myself to keep an open mind, I listened to endless stories of healing from naturopaths and other integrative medicine providers, and then I took a leap of faith when I applied this knowledge to myself—and it worked.

Now, I give you my credentials. I've already established that I am a pharmacist—the lady behind the counter in the white lab coat with a trustworthy smile. As a doctor of pharmacy (PharmD) with over eighteen years of clinical experience, I proudly hold expertise in many medication-related topics and possess a well-rounded résumé that includes hospice, pain management, critical care, anticoagulation services, cardiac ICU care, diabetes, home infusion, and retail pharmacy management. A majority of my clinical experience was spent working as a hospital inpatient clinical pharmacist. Driven by a desire to further my expertise and to carve a unique subspecialty,

I developed a niche medication safety program for a three hundred plus-bed hospital, retaining the title of medication safety officer for four years. My special talent remains the uncanny ability I have to find a needle in the haystack when investigating drug-related events. Details other professionals often miss, I will likely find. I was a CSI pharmacist—a hybrid, modern-day Sherlock Holmes meets Nancy Drew, a true detective, if you will. I thrived on the process of discovery, searching for clues and assembling pieces of very complex medication-related puzzles. Most of my time was spent hunched over my computer scanning reports, generating data, combing medical records, and presenting detailed patient safety summaries at multiple hospital committee meetings. It was my job to protect the staff, to keep the patients safe from harm, and to create safety systems that would prevent repeat events. Even with the best intentions and the best technological systems money can buy, adverse drug events, like medication errors and adverse drug reactions, happen every single day, in every single hospital in this country.

With several years of clinical experience under my belt and a desire to pad my résumé (and grow my 401[k]), I took my expertise on the road when I landed a job as a medical liaison with the pharmaceutical industry. During the next four years, I wholeheartedly believed I was providing a valuable educational service to fellow health care providers, under the guise of medical education. I was oblivious to the fact that I was causing harm by providing another cog in the well-oiled pharma wheel. Eventually, circumstances led to an *aha* moment, when I realized I was merely a glorified sales rep with a fancy title. Once I became more aware of the role I was playing, I found I had to force myself to lower my ethical standards on a daily basis each time I was reciting twisted half-truths taught to me by masterfully crafted drug resources. I was part of the problem. How could a pharmacist who practiced with integrity, trust, and compassion get stuck in the sticky pharma web of deceit? Clever trickery was in play, the same art of manipulation used on health care providers every single day—bought with impressive sales slicks, an expensive deli sandwich, and free medical education or, in my case, an impressive compensation package and perks galore.

Paralleling with the time span I worked for pharma, I experienced some of my greatest personal health challenges. By the grace of God, and a stroke of good luck, I was divinely directed into the world of functional medicine. In 2011, I completed a natural medicine fellowship and obtained board certification through the American Academy of Anti-Aging and Regenerative Medicine (A4M). This knowledge base provided me with the skills necessary to successfully navigate my own medication regimen and, ultimately, seek the root cause of my ailments. A double whammy education in both traditional and holistic medicine provided me with the expertise required to safely dissect my medication regimens and lifestyle practices, so I could slowly remove most of my drug therapies and begin the road to healing and recovery. I became an integrative pharmacist, or a functional pharmacist. I now possess knowledge in the following complementary and functional approaches to medicine—nutrition, herbals, supplements, medicinal foods, detoxification, health coaching, motivational interviewing, and compounding pharmacy. I adhere strictly to treating disease with a trifecta that encompasses a focus on mind, body, and spirit. Optimal health cannot be achieved if one of these elements is missing. Every day, I apply analytical skills to recognize drug-drug interactions, drug-herb interactions, and drug-nutrient depletion disorders. I work with the patient and health care provider to offer solutions in a team approach that encourages each patient to assume individual responsibility for his or her own health choices, thereby improving overall quality of life. I adhere to the oath "do no harm" and hold patient safety, efficacy of therapies, and the appropriate use of evidence-based information to the highest regard. I treat the patient as a whole person by utilizing a holistic approach to the delivery of quality care and am versed in prevention, wellness, and lifestyle modalities. My mission is ultimately to provide you with "health care," not "sick care," and to hone in on your body's amazing ability to heal itself.

At present, I work in a retail pharmacy setting. As part of my continuous learning mission, I have tasked myself with understanding all aspects of my profession. In order to slay the beast, one must get inside it to find how it thrives and survives. I am witnessing more and more dissatisfied patients who are seeking alternatives to expensive and toxic drug therapies. I have positioned myself on the front line and possess a unique opportunity to positively impact the well-being of many lives. Negative media and fake news flood the airwaves daily, leaving most consumers confused about health topics and searching for a trusted, reliable, and respected professional opinion. I have dedicated myself to this task and am willing to take a personal and professional leap of faith to educate you and offer better healing solutions. If pharmaceutical drugs are the problem, then staying healthy is the solution. *Undrugged* exposes the truth, free of bias and pharma-driven propaganda. I walk the walk and talk the talk and now live my life *undrugged*—and you can too.

Life is Better *Undrugged*

I discovered, and soon you will too, that life is simply better *undrugged*. This book is an empowering catalyst to give you the necessary knowledge and instill confidence in your ability to embark on a personal healing journey. Once you become more aware of a drug's myriad collection of health-impairing issues, you will be more motivated to remove the drug insult, identify and correct the problem's root cause, and ultimately replace the drug with safer natural solutions. You will soon realize that your health choices have been unfairly influenced by clever pharma propaganda and drug data wizardry, resulting in a destructive drug path riddled with long-term consequences and safety threats precipitated by disturbing side effects, interactions, drug-induced diseases, and nutrient depletions.

Undrugged Sleep is broken into two distinct sections to address the problems and to offer viable solutions, thus solidifying the need for an *undrugged* life. In Part I, I expose sleep drug-related issues and question whether the drugs themselves actually contribute to worsening sleep issues. I then introduce you to current FDA-approved insomnia drugs, give a brief sleep drug history, and offer a glimpse into pharma's role in turning insomnia into a medical problem. I will dispel, or confirm, myths regarding the efficacy and safety of the Z-drugs in chapter 4, "The Truth About Z-Drugs: A Pharmacist's Synopsis." Particularly interesting are the "zolpidem zombie" side effects—sleep driving, sleep eating, sleepwalking, sleep talking, and even sleep sex, along with interesting lawsuits using the "zolpidem defense." Finally, I will present the potential and crucial, nutrient-depleting *unvitamin* effects contributing to the creation of drug-induced diseases.

Part II of *Undrugged Sleep* provides you with practical and simple natural solutions to eradicate your sleep woes without resorting to potentially harmful drug therapy. I will give you several drug-free, natural medicine alternatives for eradicating insomnia. Before you can heal from any possible drug-related damages, the offending drug needs to be removed. I offer suggestions to help navigate drug removal and then guide you into a reverse and recover phase. Several lifestyle modifications and tips for healthier habits are included. Drugs, supplements, and herbs that *cause* insomnia are covered, as well as suggestions for insomnia drug alternatives using nutraceuticals, herbs, and aromatherapy. In addition, I give suggestions for sleep-boosting, nutritious food alternatives, as well as foods to avoid that hinder sleep and contribute to insomnia.

When you finish this book, I know you will embrace a "no Band-Aid" approach to healing and achieving optimal health. *Undrugged* is your catalyst to restoring rejuvenating rest that will have you sleeping like a baby in no time. I offer you *Undrugged* as a truly drug-free solution to ineffective, shortsighted, and imperfect pharmaceuticals and medical care.

PART I

Are Sleep Drugs Worsening Your Insomnia?

CHAPTER 1

Insomnia: A Medical Indication in Need of a Drug

> Once upon a time, drug companies promoted drugs to treat disease. Now it is often just the opposite. They promote diseases to fit their drugs.
>
> —Marcia Angell, MD, former editor in chief of the *New England Journal of Medicine* and author of *The Truth about Drug Companies*

We live in a "take a pill and go to sleep" era. Like Pavlov's dogs, insomnia-plagued Americans have been trained to pop a pill to reap a sleep reward, expecting to immediately fall asleep and stay asleep, with little or no effort. It is the path of least resistance, giving us an easy-way-out option, rather than confronting the root cause of our insomnia. Just "set it and forget it" so we can discretely walk away from our responsibility to identify our own underlying issues. Knowing this, it should come as no surprise that 25 percent of Americans take insomnia medications every year.[1] Twenty years ago, Ambien (zolpidem) was introduced to the market—hailed as the supposed solution to all of our sleep complaints. Ambien belongs to a category of sleep agents called Z-drugs, originally promising to provide us with a safer alternative to benzodiazepines without a hangover effect or overdose potential. Z-drugs quickly became widely overused, and many consumers fell victim to the increased risk of addiction. Yes, you and I got hooked; according to a 2013 analysis published by the Addiction Center, over nine million Americans routinely use sleeping pills and 30 percent are dependent. With up to seventy million Americans using sleeping pills today, the CDC (Centers for Disease Control and Prevention) has even deemed insufficient sleep as a *public health epidemic*.[2]

The situation seems to have gotten out of hand, allowing the thief of sleep to prevail by effectively stealing our precious rest and forcing us to install a drug-based security system. When did synthetic chemicals become the primary chosen defense? The story gets far more interesting. From 1993 to 2007, the United States witnessed a sevenfold increase in new insomnia cases, corresponding with an astounding *thirtyfold increase* in Z-drug prescriptions.[3] From 1999 to 2010, office visits for sleep-related complaints increased by 30 percent, demonstrating that Americans were being plagued by an insomnia *epidemic*. To keep up with the feverish pace of new insomnia diagnoses, new sleeping pill prescriptions exploded in volume from 5.3 million in 1999 to *20.8 million* in 2010—an increase of 290 percent over ten years, dominated by a mind-boggling 350 percent increase in Z-drugs alone.[4] Coincidentally, or maybe not, a pharma-driven, aggressive insomnia awareness campaign strategically paralleled Z-drug market launches, beginning with zolpidem (Ambien) in 1993. Over a fifteen-year span, Z-drug prescriptions were being dispensed twenty-one times more rapidly than verified diagnoses related to sleeplessness and five times more rapidly than insomnia diagnoses. Basically, physicians became vending machines for sleep candy. It is blatantly clear, excessive Z-drug prescriptions were being written daily without corresponding documented medical indications.[5] Something smells rotten—is it genius marketing or mastery in the art of manipulation?

After dedicating years of my life to clinical pharmacy practice, I realized that an insomnia epidemic didn't suddenly appear out of thin air. It was created by a pharmaceutical industry-spawned marketing tactic called "disease mongering." Disease mongering extends the boundaries of treatable illness and expands the market for new products.[6] In essence, sickness is sold to boost the booming business of drugs and devices. But exposed to the light of day, this is really nothing more than creating drugs that are in search of an indication. Pharma convinces healthy people that they are unwell and the slightly unwell to think they are gravely ill and then persuades them that everyone requires drug treatment. For instance, shyness is now "social phobia";

kids simply being normal, energetic kids now have "attention deficit hyperactivity disorder (ADHD)"; and 10 percent of the population is now affected by restless leg syndrome (RLS), a "disease" warranting, yes, yet another drug.[7]

Even before officially launching Z-drugs, pharma masterminded an ambitious insomnia educational campaign intending to prime the medical community. Under the guises of public service awareness, practitioners, including myself, and consumers were shrewdly targeted to begin questioning personal sleep habits and overall sleep quality and quantity. Once the stage was set for a groundbreaking unmet need, pharma sold the promise that a mere little pill could guarantee a good night of restful sleep, followed by a productive day. After questioning individual sleep needs, enticing ads followed with, "Sleep the night and seize the day ... A better tomorrow begins tonight," and, "Does your restless mind keep you from sleeping?" Like a fairy godmother granting wishes and dangling glass slippers, pharma offered a magical solution—one Americans eagerly believed and, thus, quickly bought what drug companies were selling. Even with years of medical education and drug expertise, I had the wool effectively pulled over my eyes—I bought what they were selling. I allowed the power of influence to dupe me into believing my ailments required pharmaceutical intervention.

Today, the odds of achieving blockbuster drug status are rare, requiring over $1 billion in annual sales. As a practicing pharmacist, I personally witnessed when pharma struck gold in 2006, achieving blockbuster status with Z-drugs and earning manufacturers $3 billion in combined drug sales for zolpidem and eszopiclone. To hit the mark, pharma invested heavily in direct-to-consumer (DTC) marketing, spending $850 million in 2006 and another $500 million in 2007, yielding an additional four million prescriptions.[8] New insomniacs continued to be diagnosed in America, and the sleeping pill trend steadily increased by 60 percent from 2000 to 2010, with over 4 percent of adults taking sleep aids at least once a month.[9] Much Z-drug marketing has since halted due to patent expirations and sales being dominated by generics. However, newer sleep agents are generating a resurgence of ads, once more attempting to appeal to your emotions.

Do you question whether you've been unfairly influenced by pharma advertising? A cause and effect phenomena can be postulated, whereby disease mongering effectively generated a paradigm shift in

Dr. Lori Arnold, PharmD

insomnia treatment. Unfortunately, the pendulum swung in the wrong direction. Prior to the inception of pharmaceutical sleep agents, we relied on herbs and food as primary treatment for sleep issues. Agents like melatonin and chamomile were widely utilized, along with relaxation techniques. Recently, pharma entered the natural medicine marketplace by introducing a prescription-only version of melatonin, a supplement backed by a proven safety and efficacy track record for over a hundred years. Was pharma driven by fear of competition or desperation or even impressive profit margins when it tapped into the nutraceutical arena? We may never know the true reason.

Insomnia awareness and strategic pharma education has vastly contributed to overprescribing and overutilization of drugs as first-line treatment. Rather than calming wandering monkey minds with more cost-effective or free resourceful practices, like meditation or prayer, a trained response favors inducing a semicomatose state with the easy pill fix, designed to help you forget your worries, and then you sleep. It doesn't have to be this way. You hold the key to your personal health destiny, and every informed decision you make can bring you one step closer to improved health and increased vitality. If you want to hop on board the health train, you will need to become *undrugged*.

CHAPTER 2

Sleepless in America

> When you have insomnia, you are never really asleep, and you are never really awake.
> —*Fight Club*

I was plagued by insomnia for years. A typical night would play out much like this: I lie awake staring blankly into the darkness knowing my sleep thief has returned. My monkey mind wildly ping-pongs as I count one sheep, two sheep, three little sheep, please let me sleep. In fifteen minutes, my husband's breathing slows to a rumbling snore as he blissfully succumbs to sleep. How does he do that? I attempt to calm myself and resume my scattered counting, one sheep, two turtledoves, three French hens, Little Bo Peep, Bye Bye Blackbird. The clock mocks me at midnight, and anxiety percolates. Now infuriated with my snoozing husband, I give him a jarring shove. I hear a moment of silence, followed by a snort and resumption of the agonizing vibrato. The clock continues taunting me as I silently recite prayers, meditations, and mind-calming exercises. My body finally surrenders from exhaustion and frustration several hours later. Unfortunately, my alarm jolts me awake after only an hour, and my cheery and refreshed husband leaps out of bed. Hitting snooze, I roll over, remaining lifeless, struggling to open my eyes, disoriented, groggy, and grumpy. Unfortunately, I get to look forward to suffering brain fog and another unproductive day while I begin to prematurely dread tonight's encore. This is insomnia.

Dr. Lori Arnold, PharmD

Sleepless in America is not a Meg Ryan and Tom Hanks movie. This is real-life drama fueled by performance anxiety keeping you up all night worrying about being up all night. If you battle nightly dream stealers, you are one of the fifty to seventy million American adults with chronic sleep disorders.[10] If a more persistent pattern develops, forcing you to seek medical attention, you join 10 percent of Americans with clinically diagnosed insomnia.[11] Insomnia follows acute or chronic patterns of sleepless nights with difficulty *falling* asleep, *returning* to sleep, *staying* asleep, or any combination of these. Acute insomnia is linked to stressful or devastating life events and resolves soon after the stressor is removed, usually without medical treatment. On the other hand, chronic insomnia often prompts medical intervention, exceeds three episodes a week for more than three months, and in many cases persists for two or more years.[12]

Prolonged sleep deprivation may force you into an active nocturnal existence, binging on late-night exercise or cooking infomercials and marathons of *Beverly Hillbillies* and *Green Acres*. Combine this with highly charged emotions like desperation and frustration and added undesirable ill health effects, and you will find yourself primed for easy enticement by the flood of drug ads promising a simple pill solution. If you cave in, you are now one of over eight million Americans using sleeping pills to maintain a good night's rest.[13] For many, effortlessly popping a pill beats adjusting sabotaging habits in order to eliminate the sleep thief. If you are part of the sleeping-pill nation, as I was, or are searching for ways to avoid joining this group, this book is for you.

Sleep Is a *Luxury*, Not a Priority

Optimal daytime functioning requires rejuvenating sleep, but somehow society has shifted sleep from a priority to a *luxury*. American's total sleep time has decreased 20 percent over the last one hundred years. This substantial sleep loss originates to a literal light bulb moment that happened on December 31, 1879. On this date, Thomas Edison unleashed the long-lasting incandescent light bulb on the world, and it quickly became the most sleep-disruptive invention ever.[14] By 1914, Edison identified sleep as a "bad habit," officially declaring sleep as optional and chiding that, without forced darkness, there is no reason to sleep at all. Today, with light available twenty-four hours a day plus compact, techy gadgets and gizmos entertaining us in bed, together with a barrage of self-inflicted scheduling obligations, we've morphed into busybodies too distracted to succumb to primal sleep needs.

Constant sources of mental stimulation create a never-ending pursuit of ways to energize and fuel our bodies with more caffeine, nicotine, and sugar so we can work harder, faster, and more effectively to create bigger, better, and more fulfilling lives. For many on a quest to achieve their personal best and running tandem with Edison's reprimanding sleep remarks, sleep takes backseat to a millionaire-guru mind-set of "I can sleep when I'm dead." A high-strung, stressed-out, fast-paced life effectively depletes an already dismal sleep budget. Skimping on sleep carries a lofty price tag payable in exorbitant health-burden costs. Eventually, it *will* catch up with you. Maya Angelo said it best: "When you know better, you do better." I am certain this is the reason why many opt for the sure-thing drug solution to counteract known poor habits and excessive daytime stimulation.

Burning-the-candle-at-both-ends, stressful lifestyles hail as the chief cause of insomnia. Pinpointing the source of the sleep disruption, whether environmental, lifestyle-induced, or even related to a medical condition, will provide valuable information. If you enlist a skilled sleep disorder practitioner to evaluate emotional or physical causes who won't automatically scribble a script for a sleeping pill, you will discover underlying physical dysfunctions that are not obvious. For instance, nighttime spasms and sporadic leg movements may be restless leg syndrome (RLS). Of course, pharma now has a drug for that, but RLS doesn't always require drug treatment. Natural RLS solutions are effective if the condition is caused by nutrient deficiencies, electrolyte imbalances, or even drug reactions. For some, slumber interruption stems from a physically active *parasomnic* dream state allowing one to kick, talk, or scream. This reaction is similar to a puppy whimpering, yipping, or even chasing rabbits in his sleep. That's all adorable and nonthreatening. However, in the human world, some spouses have been punched, smacked, slapped, or seriously injured while the agitated sleeper defends him or herself from a dream attacker. Some sleep disruptions are caused by the sensation of choking, gasping for breath, or even dreaming that you are drowning or being smothered. You may have stopped breathing due to obstructive sleep apnea (OSA), which contributes to sleep fragmentation and excessive daytime drowsiness. Other sleep disrupting medical conditions include chronic pain, Alzheimer's and dementia, benign prostatic hypertrophy (BPH), hormonal issues like menopause, heart disease and arrhythmias, diabetes, lung diseases like COPD and asthma, digestive issues like acid reflux (GERD) and irritable bowel, depression, attention deficit disorder, anxiety, panic disorder, and substance abuse.

Sleep Deprivation Is Disastrous

Sleep deprivation is highly dangerous. It can lead to devastating consequences and has been implicated in numerous horrific public disasters. For instance, operator fatigue due to lack of sleep was responsible for grounding the Exxon Valdez and for the nuclear meltdown at Three Mile Island, in addition to an estimated one hundred thousand motor vehicle accidents related to driver fatigue and excessive drowsiness, according to the US National Highway Traffic Safety Administration.[15] These tragic incidents demonstrate the massive toll long-term sleep deprivation takes on your mind, body, and daily functioning.

Skimping on sleep mimics an immune response similar to stress or disease, explaining why you often feel physically sick after a restless night. This launches a zombie-like *walking dead* chain reaction that has you dragging yourself through the day sluggish, fatigued, drowsy, disoriented, and anxious. Your brain may be plagued by a fog, adversely affecting your memory, cognition, concentration, problem-solving ability, and mood. Piggyback everything with indigestion, headaches, and pain.[16] Imposing these adverse effects on yourself will have you wishing you could crawl back into bed for a do over.

A continued insomnia pattern will set the stage for a perfect storm with a tsunami of symptoms that throw your body into full-blown fight-or-flight crisis mode. The harmonious hormonal symphony responsible for controlling stress, appetite, and rejuvenation is now compromised. Elevated stress hormones, like cortisol and adrenalin, encourage the body to store fat, thereby promoting obesity, heart disease, and diabetes. Unbalanced appetite-controlling hormones such as leptin and ghrelin intensify fat and carbohydrate cravings, leading to snack attacks and late-night binge eating. Finally, crucial restorative hormones responsible for cellular renewal and regeneration, like growth hormone and melatonin, are severely depleted, placing you on a road to accelerated aging. Sleep is fundamental to rejuvenate, repair, and remain youthful, so reject the pharmaceutical Kool-Aid and advice from any guru who preaches, "You can sleep when you're dead." In the quest to be my personal best, I have been guilty of following an entrepreneur's mind-set, which creates massive results by overextending working hours and, subsequently, robs time that should be reserved for sleep. Heeding misguided advice and de-prioritizing sleep in order to accomplish other tasks may just make you a sacrificial lamb; you'll never enjoy the rewards of your sacrifices if you are buried six feet under.

Without hesitation, sleep needs to be a priority, not a luxury; therefore, you need to get more of it. The *undrugged* insomnia solutions provide many useful ways to reunite you with your long-lost sleep relationship so you can dream about sheep, not count them. Before jumping ahead of myself, I want to give you a clear understanding of why sleeping pills need to be removed from your insomnia battle plan. Is it possible that sleeping pills actually steal your sleep, causing more damage than good? I will let you be the judge.

CHAPTER 3

Trouble Sleeping? We Have a Drug for That

The best doctor gives the least medicine.
—Benjamin Franklin

Drugs Used for Insomnia (FDA-Approved)

Z-hypnotics, Z-drugs, non-benzodiazepines: zolpidem (Ambien, Ambien CR, Edluar, Intermezzo, Zolpimist); eszopiclone (Lunesta), zaleplon (Sonata)
benzodiazepines: flurazepam (Dalmane), quazepam (Doral), triazolam (Halcion), estrazolam (Prosom), temazepam (Restoril)
melatonin agonists: ramelteon (Rozerem), tasimelteon (Hetlioz)
orexin antagonists: suvorexant (Belsomra)
H1 antagonists: doxepin (Silenor)
off-label sleep drugs: trazodone (Desyrel), amitriptyline (Elavil), gabapentin (Neurontin), mirtazapine (Remeron), quetiapine (Seroquel)
over-the-counter sleep drugs: all agents containing diphenhydramine (Benadryl) or doxylamine (Unisom)

History

For centuries, insomnia has been the notorious sleep thief tormenting and robbing us of one of life's most precious treasures, sending us on an endless hunt to capture an elusive dream-inducing solution. In ancient times, people attempted to force sleep by consuming herbs, smoking opium, and drinking themselves silly. Opium and alcohol remain poor options, however. Natural herbal solutions were unfortunately replaced with synthetic pharmaceutical sleep aids in the 1800s. Since then, pharma has been on an endless pursuit to engineer a safer and more effective pill.

In 1869, chloral hydrate became the first documented chemical sleep aid. Though efficient at knocking people out, it had wicked side effects and a narrow safety window between being effective and causing accidental overdose. Basically, you could either fall asleep or you could die. The options were limited, and the risk far exceeded the benefit. Adding insult to injury, tolerance developed within a few days of use, prompting many to attempt dose escalation to maintain the same effect. If you surmised this would cause more deaths from unintentional overdose, you would be correct.

In the early 1900s, barbiturates were launched, boasting safety improvements. Multiple benefits helped barbiturates gain enormous popularity, and soon many were using these agents for sleep, anxiety, psychiatric conditions, and to control socially unruly people. By World War II, Americans seeking solace from war-related stress were consuming over a billion barbiturates annually. Pegged as "downers," these agents and their use soon became synonymous with addiction and abuse, leading some psychologically unsound people to discover suicide could be successfully accomplished by downing a bottle of pills. America's most famous overdoses included Marilyn Monroe, Judy Garland, and Jimi Hendrix. Today, pentobarbital (a barbiturate) is an agent used in the lethal dose cocktail for execution of death row inmates.[17] Once again, pharma's improved agent proved too risky when used inappropriately or irresponsibly.

The 1960s, known for sex, drugs, and rock 'n' roll; free love; and hippies, also ushered in the next best safe and effective sleep agents, the benzodiazepines. Launched in 1963, diazepam (Valium) dominated the insomnia market for over a decade, from 1969 to 1982. Coined "mother's little helper," diazepam mixed with a strong martini

Dr. Lori Arnold, PharmD

pacified a generation of bored and frustrated suburban housewives. If it sounds too good to be true, it probably is. Again, safety concerns erupted with emerging overdoses and dependence, especially in combination with alcohol and other depressants. Anna Nicole Smith's infamously publicized suicide in 2007 was successfully executed with an eleven-drug cocktail containing four different benzodiazepines mixed with seven other drugs. The menacing, imperfect, and hazardous benzodiazepine safety profile challenged pharma to return to the lab once more.

America financially prospered during the 1990s. Innovation and technology boomed with advances in mobile phones, personal computers, and the birth of the World Wide Web. We were introduced to hip-hop music, *Harry Potter*, and *Seinfeld*. The quiet little chain of coffee shops, Starbucks, exploded onto the scene, adding over 2,400 shops nationwide—creating our caffeine addiction and coffee obsession. A profitable economy invited pharma to revisit gaps in unmet needs for sleeping agents. In 1992, the non-benzodiazepine drug class, known as Z-hypnotics or Z-drugs, launched with zolpidem (Ambien). We quickly fell under a spell, enticed by marketing promises that we'd fall asleep faster, without morning grogginess or next-day hangovers. A unique mechanism specifically targets the GABA-A (gamma-aminobutyric acid) receptor, allowing Z-drugs to induce sleep by slowing brain activity. Original company-sponsored research claimed Z-drugs were safer and more effective than benzodiazepines. However, recent evidence contradicts these claims. As a result, formularies written by several international regulatory groups, including NICE (the National Institute of Clinical Excellence, a European health authority), now preferentially select benzodiazepines over Z-drugs.[18]

According to *Consumer Reports Best Buy Drugs*, when compared to those not taking sleeping pills, the average Z-drug user fell asleep only eight to twenty minutes faster and gained a mere three to thirty-four minutes more sleep time. According to these unimpressive findings, I find it nearly impossible to justify taking the risk involved with using Z-drugs. After twenty plus years of actual patient use under normal, uncontrolled circumstances, significantly more data has been compiled on the ever-expanding Z-drug side effect profile, as I will cover later in this chapter.

The early 2000s continued the streak of technological advances, introducing high-speed internet, text messaging, and social media—we officially became selfie obsessed. We got caught up in reality television like *American Idol* and *The Bachelor*. *Avatar* topped the box office, *global warming* became a household phrase, and diseases dominated media attention, frightening us with threats of H1N1, SARS, and MRSA. This era became especially fruitful for pharma industry, with an explosion of television and internet drug marketing and steadily increasing drug prices. Acknowledging emerging issues and looming patent expirations with Z-drugs, pharma shifted focus to developing drugs targeting melatonin receptors, the melatonin agonists. Melatonin is a hormone and antioxidant made in the brain and GI tract that helps regulate the body's internal clock. Some forms of insomnia have been linked to melatonin depletion, thereby helping pharma justify the creation of a drug that keeps internal melatonin at normal levels. Ramelteon (Rozerem) was approved in 2005, followed by tasimelteon (Hetlioz) in 2014.[19] Because melatonin supplements are available without a prescription, controversy erupted when consumers questioned the motive behind introducing a higher-priced prescription-only version. Pharma quickly responded by boasting that the chemical version of melatonin worked longer, was more effective for sleep-onset issues, and was far superior to supplements due to lack of FDA-regulation and oversight of supplement efficacy and purity. They also emphasized the need to discourage patient self-treatment of insomnia, thus reestablishing physician supervision of treatment. I would be remiss not to mention pharma also exaggerated the exceptional benefit gained by having insurance plans cover partial costs, thus defraying 100 percent out-of-pocket expense. To simplify, pharma tried to convince each patient that, somehow, the prescription version was saving more money. What is the actual cost savings when, in early 2017, a one-month supply of ramelteon 8 mg cost an astounding $420, or nearly $14 per tab? Pharma's justifications are flimsy at best. Many manufacturers produce high quality over-the-counter nutraceutical-grade supplements, conduct independent research, and voluntarily submit purity data to the FDA. For years, I have placed my trust in many reputable nutraceutical companies, faithfully purchasing and recommending high-quality supplements to my clients. In fact, I obtain my personal nutraceutical regimen from many of these same sources. As a clinician, I do not stand alone in my stance against the use of a prescription melatonin. The European Committee for Medicinal Products for Human Use (CHMP) published a negative ramelteon review, showing an unfavorable risk-benefit balance, essentially confirming more side effects were seen with use of the prescription agents.[20]

The newbie of sleeping agents, suvorexant (Belsomra), was approved in 2014. By blocking orexin A and orexin B receptors in the brain, this drug mimics narcolepsy, which is a condition characterized by sudden and uncontrollable bouts of deep sleep. Unfortunately, due to the newness of this agent, post-marketing safety data is scant, and the full scope of side effects remains to be seen. Due to adverse effects data from pre-marketing drug studies, some experts are concerned patients may experience an increase in cataplexy, which is sudden loss of muscle tone and an increase in energy and excitation. These effects are completely opposite of the sleep-inducing effect insomniacs are striving to achieve.[21] Several more orexin-targeting agents are in the development pipeline hoping for market launch in the near future. As long as consumers keep demand for sleeping pills high, pharma will continue expanding the market by creating more new treatments, without ceasing their quest for the bigger, better, and most profitable blockbuster agent.

CHAPTER 4

The Truth About Z-Drugs: A Pharmacist's Synopsis

> You can't afford to get sick, and you can't depend on the present health care system to keep you well. It's up to you to protect and maintain your body's innate capacity for health and healing by making the right choices in how you live.
> —Dr. Andrew Weil

What do you *hope* to achieve by taking a sleeping pill? This sounds like a "duh" question; you want sleep. I know I was desperately trying to achieve hours of productive sleep while I was taking sleep aids. You and I *hope* we will achieve a blissful state of restful and rejuvenating sleep. You and I *hope* we will reap the benefits of a rested night by being able to work better, think better, and function better the next day. You and I *hope* that prescription sleep aids will be a temporary fix and will not result in long-term use or dependence. Expectations and actual experiences may vastly differ, often yielding more disappointing results than anticipated.

Z-drugs are the wolf in sheep's clothing. Governing bodies require research proving the safety and effectiveness of all drugs in order for them to gain FDA approval. It is this research that provides the framework for each drug's package insert—that multiply-folded, comprehensive document included with each drug that details all premarketing drug data and is printed in less than eight-point font requiring a magnifying lens to decipher and is far too daunting for most individuals outside the medical profession to tackle. Once a drug is granted FDA-approval, it can be released to the market, thus allowing consumers like you and I to reap the benefits of these chemical innovations. Time is money, and pharma desires an efficiently streamlined and seamless approval process in order to blanket physicians' offices with their robust sales force as quickly as possible. Even though the market launch of Z-drugs was successfully accomplished without a hitch, over time, cracks formed in the not-so-perfect foundation, once more exposing mounting cases of patient harm and heightened safety concerns. Did pharma fall short on the many marketed sleep promises? I will let you decide for yourself after examining the good, bad, and ugly—accurate and unbiased Z-drug evidence and facts.

The Good

To pass the rigorous drug approval process, Z-drugs *must have* demonstrated an element of "good." In sleep innovation, pharma often says, "We have a drug for that." If you can't fall asleep immediately after your head hits the pillow, we have a drug for that. If you can't sleep an entire night uninterrupted, stop fretting; we have a drug for that. If you wake often and can't fall back asleep, don't worry; we have a drug for that. If you suffer from a combination of issues, no problem; we have a combination of drugs for that. I think you get the idea.

Many people still swear they *feel like* they achieve better sleep with Z-drugs versus taking nothing at all. We have no way of knowing if the pill improved sleep, if sleep habits have been modified, if the situation that induced insomnia have been resolved, or if it was merely placebo effect. For many, it is highly appealing to fall asleep quickly and effortlessly by swallowing a pill and going to bed. Many people claim they benefitted from short-term use of Z-drugs, affirming one or two doses helped reset normal sleep patterns. Those with erratic and unpredictable sleep patterns—like jet-lagged travelers who need to adjust to various time zones or induce sleep during extensive international flights or shift workers who need to sleep during the day—often rely on Z-drugs. Some people suffering from nighttime awakenings depend on a low-dose, shorter-acting pill to fall back asleep more easily. Finally, for many with decent prescription drug coverage, cost may no longer be a factor, with the availability of generic equivalents, thus making a drug sleep solution more accessible and affordable.

To discourage insomnia self-treatment, well-intentioned doctors prescribe these agents, assuming the additional medical guidance and continued follow-up will give them the ability to track treatment progress, thus improving patient safety. Unfortunately, in many instances, this is not the case, and I have seen countless patients inappropriately being prescribed Z-drugs long-term, at high doses unapproved by the manufacturer and FDA and, ultimately, using Z-drugs continuously with multiple recurring refills that do not require a physician follow-up visit. In the retail pharmacy setting, it only requires a pharmacist-initiated call to a physician's office for a refill, and voilà, the patient is able to continue uninterrupted treatment. Safety-wise, Z-drugs are an improvement over older agents, like chloral hydrate and barbiturates. Chemical modifications that led to the creation of Z-drugs significantly decreased overdoses, with a higher incidence of toxicities seen when paired with alcohol and/or other depressants. Evidence also confirmed less addiction potential when compared to older agents. When compared to diphenhydramine, known for lingering grogginess, hangover effects, confusion, constipation, dry mouth and urinary retention, the shorter-acting Z-drugs proved superior with the added bonus of an improved side effect profile.

My summation highlighting positive remarks makes Z-drugs sound pretty good, right? You may be nodding in agreement, believing that Z-drugs are, in fact, advantageous for insomnia treatment. Given what I've told you up to this point, a logical assumption favoring Z-drugs might be made. However, there are two sides to every coin so let's flip this coin and see what appears on the "bad" side.

The Bad

We all wanted to believe Z-drugs were our perfect little sleeping pill. It was inevitable that the original favorable claims would fall short and disappoint, souring the situation for drugmakers and consumers alike. Something bad was lurking in the shadows. A conundrum of concerning safety issues and less-than-stellar efficacy data should soon have you second-guessing your first-choice insomnia treatment.

What's the big deal? If a Z-drug works for sleep, why not leave well enough alone? The first and most obvious reason is that pills don't

Dr. Lori Arnold, PharmD

"cure" insomnia. Like many pharmaceutical drugs, Z-drugs offer a quick solution without addressing the actual root cause of sleeplessness. If your nightly routine includes downing a pill to induce sleep, you should instinctively ask "why" your body isn't succumbing to sleep on its own. A comprehensive sleep and lifestyle assessment may be long overdue if you haven't done one thus far. By scratching below the surface and digging a little deeper, you may unmask untreated issues like stress or depression or overlooked physical issues like apnea and hormonal imbalances.

Next, when you and I take a drug for sleep, we feed pharma's desire to sell us more drugs, thereby keeping us trapped as drug drones on a hamster wheel. If you are desperate for sleep, you may be considerably more vulnerable to believe whatever experts in the field are telling you. Unfortunately, pharma-supplied drug information isn't always presented in a clear or trustworthy, unbiased manner, leaving much information subject to misinterpretation. Case in point—after mulling over package inserts and patient information leaflets meant to serve as the Z-drug Bible, you could be inclined to think they are safe and effective; however, these documents are wrought with bias and peppered only with positive premarketing data. By accepting pharma material at face value, you are denied a 360-degree view of the drug, which omits the most up-to-date efficacy data, along with thousands of FDA-reported and unreported cases of adverse drug reactions and omitted postmarketing safety issues. According to the fine print found in these documents, the manufacturers state that the drug will provide significant improvements in sleep latency, sleep efficiency, and overall sleep maintenance. In layman's terms, you will fall asleep faster, sleep longer, and have better overall sleep quality when compared to taking a placebo sugar pill. None of the printed material cited improvement in next-day functioning, as was highlighted in some of the original drug marketing ads.

Buyer beware—the lay public only has access to the segments of data pharma wants you to see. This constitutes an error of omission or willful blindness, which is failing to do the right thing by intentionally withholding facts that should be included. Think of it like baking. If you were mixing a cake batter and decide to omit a key ingredient like eggs, what would happen? The cake would flop, and you'd throw it away, forcing you to start over from scratch. In the world of pharmaceuticals, if important safety data or unfavorable studies are

UNDRUGGED: SLEEP

omitted intentionally or unintentionally, you may be playing Russian roulette with your life. Unlike a botched baking fiasco, an unfortunate drug incident may not afford you the opportunity for a do over.

Three distinct flaws were noted with Z-drug company-sponsored trials—publication bias, placebo comparator, and placebo response. Publication bias is a loophole allowing pharma to hand-select trials that demonstrate the most impressive safety and efficacy data. This is an incredibly important point that became a driving force for me and ultimately led to the creation of *undrugged*. I have the ability as an expert in the field of drugs to utilize my discerning eye to uncover the truth that is cleverly hidden, thereby, providing a method to get factual information to you. Here comes the whammy—when filing a new drug application with the FDA, pharma is mandated to submit all research data. However, they are under no obligation to *publish* all of the studies they conducted. Enter the "error of omission"—pharma doesn't publish what it doesn't have to. This explains why most failed, flawed, or unfavorable clinical trials never appear in printed literature. By allowing pharma the privilege of showcasing cherry-picked data, we potentially risk overestimating the actual drug effect and underestimating the safety profile. As a consequence of this negligence, physicians are being denied valuable findings they need to make appropriate and safe selections from available drug options. Instead, your physician is provided with flashy marketing-driven information courtesy of pharma reps, along with such persuasive perks as scrumptious lunches, closets bursting with free samples, and complimentary pharmaceutical education. In an attempt to combat this corrupt system, some resourceful researchers have found ways to access all of the drug data, published and unpublished. A meta-analysis study can be conducted by pooling all FDA-submitted data, including unpublished results, or researchers can perform research in a setting unfunded by pharma, like universities or governmental agencies. By utilizing these clever work-arounds, they are, in effect, uncovering and revealing the drug's truth.

"Placebo comparator" is a standard method used by pharma to gauge drug effect by comparing a group of patients taking an active drug with a group of patients taking a placebo or sugar pill, meaning a pill that has no active drug in it. Prior to FDA approval, all Z-drug manufacturer-sponsored trials utilized this method. I find this technique wishy-washy, especially since older comparator drugs, like benzodiazepines, were available to test head-to-head, offering a more accurate assessment of a drug's true effect. This clinical strategy does not seek outcomes that are best for the patient; rather, it is a business strategy that gives a new drug the best chance to glean impressive results without the risk of performing equally to or even worse than older drugs. I have reviewed many postmarketing studies that utilized a head-to-head comparison with older drugs, and the results were dismally disappointing for the newer agents, as, many times, the older agents outperformed the more expensive, newer agents. These studies are perfect examples of data the pharma industry would prefer you not see.

"Placebo response" is another identified Z-drug trial flaw. Unfortunately, this tactic leaves too much wiggle room for assumptions to be made. For instance, logically you would think taking a sugar pill devoid of active drug would not yield sleep benefits. However, this was not the case in many instances. In fact, many studies showed negligible differences between Z-drugs and placebo, thus questioning the need for a drug. How is that even possible? Subjects' insomnia may have improved with other interventions outside of drug therapy. Or perhaps it was merely the psychological effect of subjects thinking they were taking an active drug. Or finally, it may have been manipulation of statistical data when researchers estimated the difference in responses between the two subject groups, with many studies excluding more difficult to treat patients like heavy coffee drinkers (in other words, those who engaged in heavy caffeine consumption), overweight subjects, or those taking other psychotropic drugs. Not surprisingly, exclusion of these subjects can increase the potential for highly favorable results—which would be in pharma's best interest.[22]

Knowing the vast level of data manipulation used by pharma, savvy consumers hunger for bias-free and factual information. To fill that need, the Agency for Healthcare Research and Quality (AHRQ) and the National Institutes of Health (NIH) supported a comprehensive pooled data analysis from over a hundred sleep agent studies to provide accurate and nonbiased safety and efficacy information. Researchers also obtained all FDA-submitted data, published and unpublished, thereby factoring all findings into the final results.[23] Curiously, when given all the facts, NIH investigators attributed 50 percent of Z-drug response to placebo effect, leading them to conclude clinicians should be encouraging patients to focus on lifestyle and behavioral interventions before drug therapy.[24]

Now that I have established a firm background on the drugs and introduced the many sources of Pharma bias, I will focus on the performance of Z-drugs in real-life situations. Basically, how will Z-drugs perform when given to you or me at home in our normal, day-to-day routines?

Sleep Latency: How Quickly Do You Fall Asleep?

"I can't fall asleep" is an insomniac's most frequently voiced complaint. On average, those suffering from insomnia will struggle to fall asleep for over thirty minutes, wake up often during the night, and achieve less than 6.5 total hours of sleep.[25] Shooting for the moon, the original goal for drugmakers was to gain FDA-approved indications for all unmet sleep needs. After numerous failed attempts, it became clear that Z-drugs could not deliver. Therefore, pharma chose to focus on the one outcome Z-drugs impacted, sleep latency, or time it takes to fall asleep.

Pharma Promise #1. All Z-drugs help you fall asleep faster than placebo. According to manufacturer's claims, Z-drugs are superior to placebo and demonstrated statistically significant improvements in sleep latency. One drug ad posed the question, "Does your restless mind keep you from sleeping?" implying that one can calm an active monkey mind with a Z-drug.[26]

Facts. According to manufacturer's package inserts, Zolpidem (Ambien) and eszopiclone (Lunesta) outperform placebo; however, they did not furnish documentation of the actual sleep time gained. The package insert for Zaleplon (Sonata) notes chronic insomniacs fell asleep ten to twenty minutes faster than with placebo. According to the unbiased NIH study, Z-drugs may help you fall asleep within twelve minutes of your head hitting the pillow. I will put this into perspective. If it normally takes you thirty minutes to fall asleep, taking a pill may provide an extra eighteen sleep minutes. NIH found higher doses offered no additional benefit and only intensified undesirable side effects.[27] Another large-scale analysis showed Z-drugs helped subjects fall asleep within twenty-two minutes (range eleven to thirty-three minutes), with no improvements in sleep quality or total sleep time. Increasing the drug doses did result in slightly better outcomes; however, medical governing bodies no longer support high-dose therapy based on safety concerns, which ultimately led to FDA-mandated dosing revisions.[28]

When compared head-to-head with benzodiazepines, results confirmed that no additional benefit was gained by taking Z-drugs.[29] Subsequently, the 2014 American Academy of Sleep Medicine (AASM) guidelines no longer list Z-drugs as first-choice treatment for chronic insomnia.

Take-Home Message. You may fall asleep marginally faster, but it could require you to take higher unsafe doses, and Z-drugs are no longer the first-line sleep treatment choice according to experts.

Sleep Efficiency **and** *Quality:* **How Long and How Well (Perceived) Did You Sleep?**

Pharma Promise #2. Zolpidem and eszopiclone will help you sleep longer and achieve better quality sleep versus taking a placebo or no drug at all, and zaleplon did not offer additional benefit when compared to taking a placebo. According to package inserts, zolpidem and eszopiclone outcomes were superior to placebo with statistically significant improvements (meaning noticeably improved outcomes) in total sleep time, number of nighttime awakenings, and sleep quality. Achieving better overall sleep was implied by one marketing slogan that stated, "Sleep the night and seize the day ... A better tomorrow begins tonight."

Facts. According to manufacturers' package inserts, zolpidem and eszopiclone achieved sleep efficacy and quality outcomes that were better than placebo; however, actual data needed to back these claims was omitted from documents. When I scrutinized zaleplon's package insert, I was able to reveal that this drug failed to outperform the placebo group. In this case, I surmise that it is completely illogical to take a drug that works no better than a sugar pill and will plague you with a myriad of ugly side effects.

An FDA analysis revealed all Z-drugs lacked sufficient evidence to support claims that a patient will achieve improvements in sleep efficacy and quality, with most studies omitting data pertaining to these valuable sleep parameters. Looping back to an earlier point I made, once again pharma is caught cherry-picking the most favorable results in an attempt to downplay significant drug shortcomings in other valuable sleep maintenance markers.[30] If enough compelling evidence surfaces revealing a drug doesn't work as well as promised, how can I encourage providers to prescribe the drug or patients to take the drug? You judge if the pill is worth the ill, based on the following factual data addressing valid concerns with Z-drug use.

Exactly how many extra sleep minutes will you achieve by taking Z-drugs? In addition to the overblown claims of increased sleep time I have discussed, NIH showed a dismal total average sleep gain of thirty-two minutes per night.[31] A downfall to this estimate pointed out that many patients may experience skewed sleep perception due to the hypnotic action of Z-drugs—they induce amnesia, causing you to assume a false sense of quality sleep because you simply can't remember if you slept well or not. Having taken Z-drugs, I recall how hypnotic effects blurred my memory of falling asleep and dulled my recollection of nighttime awakenings. In terms of total gained sleep time per night, Z-drugs increased sleep slightly, though the negligible benefit may ultimately be trivial.[32]

Is it advisable to continue taking Z-drugs long-term? According to approved labeling, treatment duration should be, "short-term ... up to 30 days." Not one preapproval trial assessed long-term use, capping the maximum study duration at six weeks. I know from personal experience and from professional exposure as a pharmacist in the retail setting, the average real-world insomniac doesn't limit use to short-term—he or she typically pops one or more high-dose pills continuously every night for several years.[33] Some patients even feel they are doomed to lifetime treatment with these drugs for fear of rebound insomnia or worsening of sleep issues. Current 2016 American College of Physicians (ACP) Chronic Insomnia Guidelines discourage long-term Z-drug use due to lack of evidence supporting benefit and harm of sustained use. ACP also advises reassessing the patient if insomnia lasts longer than ten days. Further, ACP restricts total duration of treatment to less than five weeks.[34] In a perfect world where patients and physicians strictly adhere to Z-drug package inserts, prescriptions would be written adhering only to specific indications, meet all appropriate age and sex patient criteria, and be limited to a few intermittent days of use at the lowest effective doses. I happen to know for a fact *that* isn't happening, and safety issues associated with dose escalation and long-term use continue to soar.

Unfortunately, ACP guidelines are stricter than the FDA's stance on treatment duration. In 2005, the FDA lifted previous restrictions against long-term sleeping pill use and allowed all new sleep agents being introduced to the market at that time or in the future to include the label indication approving extended use.[35] To my disappointment, this regrettable FDA decision was based on a collection of controlled long-term studies that lasted a measly three to twelve months, with the assumption that patients were using Z-drugs sparingly rather than routinely, which you and I know hardly mimics real life.[36] I will give you a dose of real-life: Long-term Z-drug use showed 65 percent of patients exceeded 365 pills a year and took an average of 30 doses a month. Further, an alarming 33 percent of patients remained on treatment longer than five years. In another 2012 survey, 68 percent of zolpidem patients exceeded 228 doses a year, taking roughly 20 doses per month.[37] Clearly, a majority of patients take Z-drugs long-term, often continuing well past twelve months.

If taken long-term, how effective are Z-drugs over time? Study after study has confirmed that, the longer you use Z-drugs, the less effective they become. For instance, patients who took zolpidem gained an extra twenty minutes of sleep after two doses, however, by the fourteenth continuous night of use, an abysmal three minutes was gained. If that isn't disappointing enough, when compared to placebo after two weeks of use, patients reported no notable difference in sleep quality or perceived total sleep.[38] Once more, a drug that performs no better than a sugar pill—*that* is a hard pill to swallow. That is a pill I refuse to swallow.

It seems like a no-brainer to ask, if you notice your sleeping pill is not working as well as it used to, why continue taking it? Performance anxiety—stopping may be too painful. For those who have established a nightly sleeping pill routine, the fear and anxiety often associated with the repercussions of treatment discontinuation forces them to continue popping a pill whether it works or not. Eventually many of us will fall into a comfortable nightly pill habit, but could that road lead to tolerance, dependence, or even addiction? Early data showed patients taking less than fifteen doses a year did not become habituated, but clearly a majority of people far surpass fifteen doses a year. I rarely see patients utilizing sleep medication intermittently or based on infrequent circumstances prompting sleep loss. Package inserts state, "All sleep medicines carry some risk of dependency," and, "During nightly use for an extended period, tolerance or adaptation to some effects may develop." When initially introduced to the market, Z-drugs were like a shiny new car we excitedly drove off the lot. Many of us assumed we had upgraded from benzodiazepines and barbiturates, leaving undesirable tolerance, dependence, and addiction in our rearview mirror. Regretfully, the new car smell has worn off, and it is time to enact "lemon laws" due to mounting reports of Z-drug dependence, tolerance, misuse, and withdrawal symptoms.[39]

Habitually taking Z-drugs every night for several weeks creates *dependence*, a psychological dilemma that makes you think you can't fall asleep without it. In essence, we train our minds to think we cannot achieve sleep without the pill. *Tolerance* forces you to continuously increase doses to achieve the same effect, with a "sky's the limit" mentality on your final dose. In this situation, we may take a "more is better" approach without considering the consequences and find we often disregard potential safety issues and dosing limits. When people attempt to end treatment, *withdrawal*, also called rebound insomnia, frequently follows with a temporary worsening of sleeplessness that induces anxiety, abnormal dreams, nausea, upset stomach, and even hallucinations.[40] You may desire sleep without a pill but resist making a change due to the fear of the pill-detox effect. Drug companies document that withdrawal is common, lasting an average of *two nights*. Now that I have made you aware that the "pain" is common and normal and will only last a few days, and if I provide methods to appropriately taper your regimen with supportive tools, would you be more inclined to opt for safer sleep alternatives? I dare say most would opt out of drug therapy, as I have successfully done for others and myself.

Take-Home Message. Research does not support claims that Z-drugs provide refreshing, quality sleep. Though you may sleep a few extra minutes, this minuscule benefit is far outweighed by the associated alarming risks. Overriding the stance the FDA took in 2005, I stand firmly with ACP's safer recommendations discouraging long-term Z-drug use due to diminishing effects that eventually lead to unsafe dose escalations. Finally, frequently taking Z-drugs exponentially increases your risk of dependence, tolerance, misuse, and withdrawal symptoms.

Dr. Lori Arnold, PharmD

Next-Day Functioning: **Did You Perform Better the Next Day?**

Pharma Promise #3. According to marketing claims, Z-drugs carry an implied benefit of improved next-day functioning with hopeful drug ads stating, "A great night might help you become a morning person again. Wake up refreshed and recharged after a good night's sleep." **Facts**. Simply, daytime functioning is impaired, not enhanced. According to documented trials in package inserts, Z-drugs were actually confirmed to *worsen* daytime functioning and have no positive effect on performance. I would like you to consider how sleeping pills work. At bedtime, you pop a pill to halt the barrage of brain chatter and soon drift asleep as your mind and body slow down. An assumption is automatically made that all drug effects will—poof!— magically disappear the moment you open your eyes. I hate to be the bearer of bummer news, but unfortunately it doesn't work like that, as all sleeping pills have effects that linger, thus hindering next-day brain functioning.[41] This slowed brain response will plague you with daytime side effects like grogginess and disorientation, impaired learning, slowed physical movement, and impaired driving ability. The elderly often experience a myriad of these effects, plus increased confusion, memory loss, and serious falls.

Drugmakers did perform studies to verify whether Z-drugs had potential to accumulate with continued use. Unfortunately, they based all conclusions on scant seven- to fourteen-day trials. Once more, I am particularly concerned, since I know a most people use these drugs for more than fourteen days, making any results questionable and potentially misleading. The findings suggested that all drug effects "should" be gone within twenty-four hours, with the exception of the longer-lasting eszopiclone, which remains in the body for up to thirty-six hours. Note the clever use of the word "should," since no two people will experience identical drug responses. "Should be gone" does not apply if the entire drug elimination process is considerably slowed down, creating higher than normal drug levels in females, elderly, those with genetic variations or liver dysfunction, or those who are taking other sedating drugs or alcohol.

Take-Home Message. Evidence failed to support claims that you will feel better, be sharper, or have an increase in next-day performance after taking Z-drugs. Hands down, evidence proves without a doubt that Z-drugs *impair* next-day functioning.[42]

The Ugly

I hope you recall the intent of Z-drugs was to offer improved alternatives to older drugs plagued with horrible side effects and safety issues. Originally at market launch, it seemed the sleep-deprived nation's prayers were finally answered, especially when company trials showed impressive improved efficacy and safety outcomes. Today, after more than two decades of use by millions of consumers, a reliable and robust database that contains thousands of documented reports of health and safety issues is available for us to peruse. If you scratch below the surface, as I have, you will find that these drugs are not as safe as originally perceived. Z-drugs carry a major risk of harm even when used exactly as prescribed, but considerably more so when irresponsibly prescribed or inappropriately used. March on soldier—I will dive into Z-drugs' ugly side effects and complications in more detail in the next chapter.

CHAPTER 5

Side Effects and Complications: Is the Benefit Worth the Risk?

Nearly all men die of their medicines, not of their diseases.
—Moliere (1622–1673)

When contemplating getting *undrugged* from any drug therapy, you should always consider risk versus benefit. Weigh all potential risks and side effects that have potential to leave permanent damage against the consequence of suffering from a few nights of moderate sleep loss. It is certain that Z-drugs linger, causing effects that can accumulate over time. As a result, you may suffer latent grogginess and decreased awareness that could lead to more severe bodily harm. You exponentially increase health risks when Z-drugs are used in situations that heighten drug effects like liver disease, obesity, or sleep apnea or if mixed with alcohol and other sedating medications. You would be shocked by how many elderly patients tell me they take sleep medications with an evening cocktail. From what I know, removing the cocktail may actually lead to a diminished need for sleep medication, but we will get into that later. Z-drugs also significantly increase risk of serious injury from falls and are synonymous with less common amnesiac "complex sleep-related behaviors" like hallucinations, sleep eating, sleepwalking, sleep texting, sleep driving, and even sleep sex. I am going to get to this interesting phenomenon shortly, but for a majority of patients, they will more likely encounter common side effects that include:[43]

1. Headache, dizziness, and drowsiness
2. Dyspepsia, acid reflux, peptic ulcer disease, and indigestion
3. Decreased reaction time and alertness
4. Impaired learning, memory, and cognitive function
5. Slowed thought, movement, and driving ability
6. Tolerance, dependence, and withdrawal rebound insomnia with long-term use
7. Bitter, metallic taste with eszopiclone (in 35 percent of patients)

A continuously expanding side effect database has provided a wealth of information on specific Z-drug related complications, including a few that are worth detailed discussions.

Sleep Apnea

Have you ever been told that you stop breathing in your sleep? You may have sleep apnea, or uncontrollable breath pauses that occur while you sleep. Unlike a child who seeks attention by holding his or her breath, many apnea sufferers may be completely oblivious that the normal breathing reflex is compromised. Many sufferers experience vivid dreams where they feel the actual sensation of choking or drowning and find themselves struggling to awaken from freakish and frightening episodes. If unrecognized or left untreated, prolonged breathing cessation can ultimately lead to death. Elderly and obese have an apnea risk much higher than the general population.

Apnea sufferers should not take Z-drugs, as the targeted action on the GABA receptor slows down nerve response time and may cause a profound decrease in stimulation of involuntary reflexes, like breathing. If a potent unpredictable drug effect is introduced to existing lung conditions like apnea, COPD, or asthma, spontaneous breathing functions may be more difficult to restart, leading to the danger of total breath cessation. In medical lingo, it is called respiratory depression—or simply, you stop breathing. The FDA has documentation showing zolpidem worsens sleep apnea, and respiratory depression is listed in warnings and precautions. For safety reasons, experts concur, as do I, that anyone diagnosed with sleep apnea should avoid *all sleeping pills*.[44]

Dr. Lori Arnold, PharmD

Acid Reflux and Infection

Could my nighttime heartburn be caused by a sleeping pill? Say it isn't so. An association between the two is rarely made. However, once I learned the mechanism, I found it made perfect sense. This reaction falls under the notorious drug-induced disease category—once more; the pill causes the ill by increasing your risk for developing gastroesophageal reflux disease (GERD). Some experts suggest Z-drugs induce gastroesophageal regurgitation, whereby the muscular sphincter separating the stomach and esophagus relaxes too much, allowing stomach acid and contents to flow back upstream where they don't belong. Swallowing is the body's normal response to refluxing, but due to the hypnotic influence of Z-drugs, you may lose the ability to feel this irritating and unnatural sensation, which hinders the swallow reflex and leaves acidic stomach contents in the esophagus, eroding the sensitive tissue barrier for extended periods of time.[45]

Adding to the destructive insult, reduced swallowing leads to pooling of saliva and bacteria in your throat and chest, thus becoming a potential mechanism for infection that increases risk of bacterial overgrowth, upper respiratory irritation, chronic sinusitis, recurrent croup, and laryngitis.[46] No longer a theory, this infectious mechanism is backed by supporting published literature. Studies, including the manufacturer's own clinical trials, confirmed zolpidem *doubles* the risk of infectious events,[47] and all Z-drugs are associated with a 44 percent higher risk for sinusitis, pharyngitis, pneumonia, bronchitis, and influenza.[48] Further evidence revealed zolpidem was responsible for a 62 to 91 percent increase in hospitalization for serious infections[49] and significantly increased the risk of pyogenic liver abscess, a serious liver infection.[50] Higher infection risk was verified in females, elderly, and those taking high-dose therapy. Without question, there is a plentitude of supporting evidence proving Z-drugs not only cause mild upper respiratory infections, but also more severe and life-threatening infections.

Depression

I need to dispel the myth that sleeping pills help depression—sleeping pills can *cause* depression. In fact, evidence shows sleeping pills *double* the rate of new depression cases.[51] I am going to break this down in order to make some sense of this. Many people taking sleeping pills have underlying psychological issues hindering their sleep. Instead of drifting off to sleep, too often, they spend nighttime hours cycling through emotions and replaying events, keeping a busy monkey mind alert and active. Unfortunately, a pill won't fix the cause of emotional turmoil, and it is more likely to produce unfulfilling sleep, tempting you to increase the dosage for improved results. When the dose is increased beyond safe parameters, you risk sabotaging next-day functioning by inducing foggy brain and sluggish cognition, further dampening mood and ruining your day. Practice this enough, for many consecutive days or weeks, and your vicious cycle could lead to extreme measures and suicidal thoughts.

Suicide

Getting caught in an insomnia and depression cycle plays mind games in a massively destructive manner. Zolpidem use has been significantly linked to suicide in those with or without preexisting psychiatric illnesses. In fact, a 2011 pooled analysis found zolpidem *doubled the risk of suicide* or suicide attempts,[52] and when used alone or in combination with alcohol, was implicated as the causal agent in a number of suicides due to drug effects that induced irrational and unpredictable behaviors, hallucinations, and violent tendencies.[53] Sleeping drugs, in general, are associated with high suicide rates, with 30 to 40 percent of successful suicides revealing a cocktail of pills and alcohol. When combined with alcohol, the sedative and hypnotic drug effects are greatly enhanced, which then becomes deadly in the hands of those with psychological instability.[54]

Acute Pancreatitis

A flurry of safety concerns surfaced when Z-drugs were linked to an increased risk of pancreatitis. As a result, two studies were conducted showing acute pancreatitis incidence significantly increased over sevenfold with zolpidem use and doubled with zopiclone, a chemical derivative of eszopiclone.[55] Researchers in both studies stressed that considerable pancreatitis risk exists with Z-drugs and called for exercising extreme caution if Z-drug use is combined with alcohol.

Dr. Lori Arnold, PharmD

Cancer and Death

You and I would like to assume a supposed harmless sleeping pill is not linked to cancer or death, but unfortunately a flood of proof tells us otherwise. Though experts do not fully understand the cancer-causing mechanism, evidence suggests that Z-drugs are clastogenic, meaning they damage chromosomes. Destroying any part of your precious genetic code can create mutations leading to cell death or the formation of cancer cells and other abnormalities.[56]

A 2012 study assessing Z-drug use over 2.5 years found an increased risk of cancer and death. Subjects taking as little as 18 sleeping pills a year were 3.6 times more likely to die, and those who averaged over 132 sleeping pills a year had a 35 percent increased risk of developing cancer. Even more astonishing, subjects taking a total cumulative dose of zolpidem greater than 800 mg each year had a *sixfold higher risk* for death or cancer compared to subjects who did not take sleeping pills. That may sound like a lot of zolpidem, but you just need to take an average of one 5-mg dose 160 nights a year, or one 10-mg dose 80 nights a year in order to reach the 800-mg cumulative dose. Even sporadically taking a 5-mg dose only when needed for less than 30 days a year still increases your death or cancer risk *fourfold*.[57] To further support burgeoning evidence, a long-term study assessing eight years of zolpidem use found a remarkable *sixfold increase* in cancer risk among those taking at least 300 mg total cumulative doses of zolpidem per year, coupled with a considerably higher risk of death. In order to reach this yearly dose, you only need to take one 5-mg dose once or twice a week.[58] It makes me very uneasy knowing most insomniacs take much higher doses every single night for several years.

If you still have a slight inkling of doubt regarding this data, Dr. Daniel Kripke, a notable sleep expert and psychiatrist, filed a 2015 Citizens Petition to the FDA urging revision of sleeping pill warnings. He analyzed over fifty sleeping pill studies published from 2012 to 2015, verifying an increased death risk in thirty-three of thirty-four studies, with the highest risk at higher doses.[59] In my professional opinion, his assessment is very thorough and unbiased and holds considerable weight in the decision to take or not take Z-drugs. The fact remains undisputed (unless you are the pharmaceutical manufacturer)—all sleeping pills old and new, including the Z-drugs, are very dangerous.

Safety Considerations in Elderly

Elderly insomniacs face considerably more challenges than do younger counterparts with Z-drug side effects and complications due to slowed drug processing, which allows effects to linger much longer than desired. This unintended delay can create dangerous adverse effects. The American Geriatric Society (AGS) publishes the Beers Criteria, which is a list of medications the elderly need to avoid because side effect risks far outweigh any drug benefits. According to Beers, Z-drugs should not be taken daily, established geriatric dosing limits should never be exceeded, and use needs to be restricted to a maximum of ninety days due to tolerance, daytime confusion, memory problems, delirium, falls and fractures, driving impairment, and lack of efficacy.[60]

Elderly also have a significantly increased risk of falls from confusion and unsteady gait as a result of sleeping drug use.[61] As you may surmise, elderly falls are exponentially more devastating. An aged, frail body suffers more profound repercussions, such as hip fractures and traumatic brain injury, both linked to declining health and increased death. A study featured in *JAMA* analyzed over fifteen thousand nursing home residents with hip fractures and found 11 percent of these residents took a Z-drug prior to falling, resulting in a doubled risk of hip fracture from lingering drug effects.[62] In 2016, two studies found Z-drugs doubled the risk of fractures in adults older than forty years, with zolpidem accounting for nearly *tripling* the risk, prompting authors to urge extreme caution when used in all high-risk patients.[63] Yet another analysis found a two- to fivefold increase in significant side effects in elderly, affecting brain and physical functioning.[64] There is no shortage of supporting documents showing similar fall and fracture outcomes.

In 2014, The Centers for Disease Control (CDC) surveyed emergency department visits for drug events involving psychiatric medications. The investigators were shocked to discover zolpidem ranked first in adverse drug event cases, accounting for over 21 percent of ED visits in those sixty and older.[65] Finally, *British Medical Journal* published an analysis of sleeping pill use in the elderly and concluded that long-term use increased risk of cancer and death in those over sixty years of age, resulting in more harm than good.[66] A tremendous amount of evidence from many highly reliable sources confirms that Z-drug use in elderly is extremely dangerous and highly discouraged.

Zolpidem (Ambien) Facts:

- Zolpidem is the most widely prescribed sleeping pill in the United States.
- In 2013, forty million zolpidem prescriptions were dispensed to five million patients.[67]
- Zolpidem is the second most frequently dispensed psychoactive drug.[68]
- Of all zolpidem prescriptions, 63 percent are written for women.[69]
- Zolpidem is ranked first for emergency department visits for adverse effects among all psychoactive drugs,[70] and visits for zolpidem adverse reactions increased 220 percent from 2005 to 2010.[71]
- Among zolpidem patients, 34 percent also take antidepressants.[72]
- At peak marketing, name brand Ambien yielded over $2 billion in yearly sales, achieving blockbuster drug status.
- Of hospitalized patients 26 percent receive zolpidem, and 34 percent were discharged with a new zolpidem prescription, whether they needed it or not.

CHAPTER 6

Complex Sleep-Related Disorders, Parasomnias, and "Zolpidem Zombies"

> The person who takes medicine must recover twice, once from the disease, and once from the medicine.
> —Dr. William Osler

Imagine that, as part of your normal sleep routine, you pop your prescribed zolpidem and hop into bed. Your gym shoes are strategically placed by the bed, and the alarm is set for dawn. Sleep soon consumes you. Suddenly you are jolted awake, suffocating from gas fumes and gasping on blankets of billowing smoke. Excruciating pain courses through your body, and a stream of warm blood oozes down your face. Dozens of voices are shouting, screaming, even sobbing—signaling mass hysteria all around. Assuming you are having a nightmare, you desperately struggle to wake up, but quickly reality sets in when your body is overcome with burning and stabbing pain validating that this is, in fact, not just a bad dream.

A car accident has left an innocent person limp, lifeless, and lying in a pool of blood next to a mangled bicycle. Trapped in your car, the inflated airbag has you wedged between the steering wheel and the driver's seat, paralyzing any movement. The car's momentum was not hindered by impact with the cyclist; rather, a solid, massive oak tree abruptly halted it, and now your maimed car is wrapped around

Dr. Lori Arnold, PharmD

it like a crushed tin can. It's a miracle you are not dead. Still barefoot and in pajamas, you have no recollection of how, why, or where you were driving. If you survive your injuries, you are vaguely aware that life will be forever changed. Through the entire ordeal, you battle lingering grogginess and disorientation from the zolpidem dose you took two hours ago. Or was it two doses? You just can't remember.

Though I created this fictitious dramatization, several lawsuits document similar stories telling of "zolpidem zombie" blackouts. I found the stories always began with "after taking a sleeping pill" and then progresses to very serious catastrophes, where people have wrecked cars and even harmed or killed people during a drug-induced amnesic state. Not all incidents were this severe; some were just oddball bothersome behaviors, which were annoying or even humorous. Unfortunately, reports of these strange incidents still continue to pile up. After innocently taking a sleeping pill, thousands have reported falling into a lucid trance (remember these agents are hypnotics) that caused them to binge eat on late-night refrigerator raids or pizza deliveries or rack up thousands of dollars in credit card charges after crazy internet shopping sprees. One of my close friends knew when she was in a stupor because, several days later, she was bombarded with FedEx deliveries of shoes in assorted colors and styles, of course, with no recollection of online shopping. In a somnolent stupor, some people have sent unintelligible texts and emails or even left absurd, garbled phone messages. We are all warned to not drunk text. However, after taking sleep agents, we do not know what we are capable of saying. When I took zolpidem, I witnessed this on many occasions when traveling for work. My significant other had countless evening phone chats with me; however, I don't remember any of the conversations. With no memory of these nighttime episodes, many will awaken to find a bedroom full of dirty dishes, email inboxes full of weird invoices from unusual websites, or messages and voice mails from puzzled and concerned friends. Although all Z-drugs are prone to causing similar bizarre and troublesome side effects, zolpidem tops the list with the most documented incidents, case reports, and lawsuits.

Complex sleep-related disorders, also called parasomnias, are abnormal behaviors that occur while you sleep. Some of these bizarre behaviors include nightmares and night terrors, hallucinations and delusions, sleepwalking, sleep eating, sleep talking, sleep sex, and sleep driving. For several years, incidents like this flew under the radar, because most patients did not link the drug to their strange behavior, leaving thousands of instances undocumented. The situation drastically changed in 2007 after intense media coverage of the parasomnia-traffic incident connection, resulting in a staggering tenfold increase in incident reporting.[73] Today, manufacturers deny the drug and bad behavior connection by maintaining that parasomnias are rare. However, I encourage you to perform a standard internet search, and you will uncover entire websites and blogs containing hundreds, if not thousands, of personal testimonials of zolpidem-induced oddball behaviors and abnormal and outlandish incidents. As I have said, even I wasn't immune to peculiar zolpidem-induced behaviors. Fortunately, most of these effects spontaneously cease without intervention several hours after stopping zolpidem.[74] Total resolution of side effects like parasomnias happen with complete drug discontinuation—another reason to get *undrugged*.

These incidents remain grossly underreported, and I firmly believe we aren't even close to realizing the full scope of the problem. Lack of formal drug-related incident reporting to the FDA or the manufacturer creates a false assumption that a drug is much safer than it actually is. If all bloggers, physicians, and pharmacists took the extra time to file a drug-related adverse event report, I assure you, governing bodies would take notice. As it stands, casually mentioning a drug reaction to a medical professional, friend, or via social media becomes hearsay in the absence of logging a formal complaint. Adverse drug reporting is so dismal that even the Institute for Safe Medication Practices (ISMP) agrees that we need to take the FDA's MedWatch and other reports with a grain of salt due to inadequate reporting trends.

Even if you don't meet any of the high-risk criteria, zolpidem should never be considered risk-free, even at manufacturer-recommended therapeutic doses. No matter the dose, approximately 15 percent of patients will experience amnesia within twenty to thirty minutes of ingestion, blocking memory and recollection capacity.[75] Amnesia that accompanies sleep isn't too worrisome and may even be welcome to some. If you are safely sleeping in bed with a loved one, however, and start wandering around unsupervised in the middle of the night, you should be very concerned. Speaking of wandering around, it's time for a little excursion into the quirky world of real-life parasomnia episodes, interesting cases, and freakish incidents.

Dr. Lori Arnold, PharmD

Hallucinations: Pink Elephants and Unicorns

Are you seeing things? Hallucinations are uncommon, occurring in less than 1 percent of the population. Again, I believe this statistic is most likely inaccurate due to underreporting, as the episodes are brief and the amnesic effect cause many people to forget they hallucinated. The reaction is dose-dependent, meaning higher than recommended zolpidem doses result in more severe hallucinations. While most episodes are short-lived, some have reported hallucinations lasting four to seven hours. Females account for 82.4 percent of reported hallucinations, and over 50 percent of hallucinations occurred in individuals taking SSRI antidepressant drugs.[76]

Sleep Eating: The Zolpidem Binge

What? I really ate *that* while I was sleeping? Some of us have gotten a good chuckle from friends and loved ones telling stories of late-night fridge raids or detailed accounts of cooking meals while asleep. Logic cannot make sense of it, and you may have quickly deduced a laced brownie or the equivalent was involved in creating an intense case of the munchies. It may also seem completely ludicrous to use sleep eating as justification for a sudden weight gain. It's no joke—though unfathomable, this reaction is very real and happens more frequently than you think.

My most notable parasomnia involved a very disturbing sleep binge-eating food coma. For many years, I was a jet-lagged frequent business traveler. On one very unforgettable trip to Hawaii, I took zolpidem 10 mg *and thought* I was in bed, quickly drifting to sleep. A few hours later, I awoke eye-to-eye with a half-eaten chocolate protein bar on my pillow. A raging gut ache forced me to gaze downward, revealing I was the not-so-proud momma of a food baby belly. Empty food wrappers littered the hotel room. In an amnesic stupor, I ate four and a half 25-gram protein bars, two bags of popcorn, and two bags of almonds. Although I was highly disgusted and disappointed with my food binge, I became acutely more troubled by my room location on the fifty-sixth floor of a high-rise tower. I felt the ocean breeze through the wide-open deck doors, and my iPad was on a chair covered in cheesy popcorn-licked residue. The consequences of wandering around dazed, confused, and hypnotized with an unsteady gait on a tower lanai potentially could have been devastating, even fatal. One more distressing thought struck me while assessing this troublesome situation: How safe is it for a single female traveler to experience amnesic stupors in strange and unfamiliar locations? I guarantee you that it is not safe by any means; and that night went down in my history as my last dance with zolpidem, or any other prescription sleep aid. This unnerving and dangerous incident became the catalyst that forced me to seek safer sleep-inducing options for my jet lag.

Sleep eating typically occurs immediately following ingestion of zolpidem. Like a zombie, you are in a comatose state but still can physically function. Literature has found that people typically gravitate toward high-caloric food binges, like fatty or sugary foods, but a few have found themselves indulging on strange items like buttered cigarettes or whole eggs in the shell, and many travelers, like myself, have annihilated entire hotel minibars.[77] Several documented cases have found people cooking stovetop meals with their eyes half-closed, and many people have awoken to plates and food remnants in their bedrooms. As you would suspect, the victims of these incidents had not one iota of recollection except for a few binge-induced side effects like nausea, loss of appetite, and extreme fatigue. Worst-case scenario, over time, some people noticed a considerable weight gain.[78] As with most parasomnias, sleep-eating episodes cease upon discontinuation of zolpidem treatment.[79] Once I stopped prescription sleep aids and opted for nutraceuticals and better sleep hygiene, my sleep-eating episodes disappeared.

Sleepwalking: Night of the Walking Zolpidem Zombie

Somnambulism: the cool, nerdy word for sleepwalking. This fascinating phenomenon allows a sleeping individual to engage in various physical activities normally done while awake. As a result, this can potentially place a sleepwalker in numerous dangerous situations. While under the influence of zolpidem, people have committed crimes, such as thefts, or have engaged in compulsive activities like cleaning and online binge shopping. If my sleep drug caused me to pull an all-night cleaning spree while I was asleep, I probably would not be too disappointed to awaken to a sparkling clean house and the fresh aroma of bleach and Pine-Sol. Engaging in a criminal act on the other hand, not quite so pleasant.

Dr. Lori Arnold, PharmD

Zolpidem caused more sleepwalking incidents than all the other sleep aids combined. Typically, sleepwalking is a childhood disorder that occurs infrequently in adults. However, zolpidem increases adult sleepwalking risk in those who were prone to having childhood sleepwalking episodes. Basically, if you were a child bumping around in the middle of the night, knocking over knickknacks, riling the dog, and waking your parents, it is highly likely you could do it now. Unfortunately, as an adult you can get into far more trouble, especially if unsupervised. Experts postulate that stress, medication, substance abuse, and brain injury also increase your risk.[80] Sleepwalking episodes usually happen within four hours of ingestion, with a substantially increased risk if you continue taking zolpidem for greater than three months duration.[81] As with other parasomnias, the sleepwalking effect is directly related to zolpidem and, in all case reports, ceased after drug discontinuation. A final word to the wise, if you have a history of sleepwalking, Z-drugs are an unsafe option that should be completely avoided.

Sleep Driving: Drugged Driving under the Influen*zzz*

At 2:45 a.m., on May 4, 2006, Rhode Island Congressman Patrick Kennedy, son of Edward "Ted" Kennedy, crashed his car into a Capitol Hill barrier claiming he was running late for a vote—House sessions adjourned at midnight. Mr. Kennedy had no recollection of the event and blamed the incident on his nighttime Ambien dose. He served a year of probation after pleading guilty to driving under the influence of prescription drugs.

The media floodgates were opened, and soon *Dateline*, *20/20*, *60 Minutes*, and hundreds of tabloid journalists were quickly investigating a string of similar traffic-related zolpidem incidents. In 2009, there was a highly publicized case involving forty-two-year-old flight attendant Julie Ann Bronson. Upon returning from an international flight, she looked forward to enjoying a quiet night at home. After consuming five glasses of wine in three hours, she put on her pajamas, took two zolpidem tablets, and went to bed. A few hours later, she awoke panicked and disoriented in a jail cell, barefoot and still in her pajamas. Shortly after taking the zolpidem, in an amnesic stupor, she had driven her car over a mother and her two daughters, severely injuring the eighteen-month-old youngest daughter. Despite blowing two tires, she continued driving an erratic five miles on bare rims, leaving a trail of sparks and smoke. Ms. Bronson was sentenced to ten years of probation and six months of jail time. Her penance was disastrous: She lost her career, devastated a family, seriously injured a child, and has to live the rest of her life regretting this tragic night.[82] For years the association between traffic incidents and residual zolpidem effects failed to be connected, and the drugged driving phenomena quietly slipped through the cracks unnoticed. That was until the incident involving Congressman Patrick Kennedy peaked national media attention, sparking a firestorm of exposé narratives and sensational headlining news reports.

Falling asleep at the wheel is not a country song or the name of a band. This very serious parasomnia produces devastating outcomes. Zolpidem-induced, amnesic sleep driving happens in a state of confusion, decreased alertness, delayed motor skills, and irrational reasoning. Lingering drug effects are masked, creating poor judgment and a false sense of safe driving ability. Experts have coined this phenomenon "drugged driving" and further established two categories, sleep driving and drug-related driving impairment. "Sleep driving" occurs immediately following nighttime drug ingestion, during a partial arousal state of amnesia. It literally is being asleep at the wheel—a dreamlike state rendering you completely unaware of physically driving a real car. "Drug-related driving impairment" happens after awakening the following morning. Much like a hangover, this phenomenon is due to residual drug effects causing grogginess and decreased alertness.[83] Episodes of sleep driving are connected directly to the dose of drug taken and the time it was ingested. Multiple driving incidents resulted from doses exceeding 5 mg of zolpidem or 6.25 mg of zolpidem extended-release,[84] with profound driving impairment during the first four to six hours immediately following zolpidem ingestion.[85]

In March 2007, the FDA mandated firmer safety warnings on all sleeping pills; however, it wasn't enough. Tragic vehicular incidents continued to occur en masse, with a 2010 traffic fatality study finding 47 percent of drivers had tested positive for sedatives. In 2013, with over seven hundred reports of zolpidem-related impaired driving accidents on the records, the FDA finally intervened by demanding that the manufacturer of branded Ambien (zolpidem) conduct a driving simulation study to assess blood levels eight hours postdose. The results were startling, with lingering excessive drug concentrations found in 15 percent of women taking Ambien 10 mg and 33 percent of women and 25 percent of men taking Ambien CR 12.5 mg. The proof was undeniable; this study unequivocally verified residual Ambien (zolpidem) effects impaired driving and significantly increased the risk of motor vehicle accidents.[86] Based on these findings, the FDA mandated strict zolpidem dose limitations, requiring a 50 percent dose reduction on all zolpidem products. Additional FDA warnings were placed on Ambien CR (extended-release zolpidem) to avoid next-day driving for the entire day after ingestion, even if you slept a full eight hours.

Even with strict mandated dose limitations, many clinicians still do not adhere to the set limits, and prescribe outside the mandate. Working as a retail pharmacist, I get dosing alerts on a daily basis warning of excessive dosing, especially in elderly females. When I initiate a call to the physician, I am met with the same resistance time and again. "That is what the patient wants and has been taking for years. That is what they get." The only thing I can do as a responsible pharmacist is to educate the patient on the restrictions and why those rules were put in place. Again, still more justification for my *undrugged* philosophy.

Driving under the influence of Z-drugs is now mainstream and commonly known. Like screening drunk drivers for alcohol, the newest screening tests police departments utilize are capable of monitoring Z-drug levels in drugged drivers. This monitoring now affords experts the capacity to assess the impact sedative drugs have on total traffic incidents.[87] Regardless of the mounds of evidence, zolpidem and other sleep agent-related traffic incidents continue to happen. Knowledge is power; please don't let the next victim be you or your loved one.

Are You High Risk for Risky Behavior?

I assure you, Z-drugs are dangerous, and it took experts far too long to reach this conclusion. During twenty plus years of market exposure, these drugs have forged a destructive path, causing harm to countless patients. You need to protect your personal safety by knowing your own risk. Several factors can increase your sensitivity to Z-drug effects, placing you at a higher risk for odd behaviors and strange encounters.[88]

- **Female gender**: Drug levels are 45 percent higher in women versus men, especially at higher doses.[89]
- **Elderly**: Drug levels are up to 63 percent higher in elderly women versus elderly men.[90]
- **High dose**: Exceeding dose recommendations significantly increases severe drug reactions. Most incidents involved zolpidem doses over 10 mg or over 12.5 mg of the extended-release zolpidem (Ambien CR).
- **Inappropriate timing**: Taking a dose too early increases risk considerably. Most incidents occurred when the drug was taken more than an hour before bed or if the drug effect kicked in before the patient was physically in bed.
- **Combining with alcohol or other sedatives**: Manufacturers and experts *explicitly warn* that the drug effects are exponentially enhanced when combined with alcohol or other sedatives.
- **Combining with antidepressants**: Strong drug interactions between Z-drugs and SSRI antidepressants (Prozac, Paxil, Zoloft, and the like) can induce adverse psychiatric reactions. Among patients with hallucinations, 58 percent were also taking antidepressants.[91]
- **Combining with CYP P450 drugs**: Cytochrome P450 (CYP P450) enzymes affect how drugs are removed from the body. The combination could increase zolpidem concentration to toxic levels, thus enhancing drug effects and increasing side effects.
- **Malnutrition/nutritional deficiency**: Zolpidem is highly bound to serum protein; therefore, seriously ill patients or those with low serum albumin levels may experience heightened adverse effects.
- **Living alone**: Living alone vastly increases risk for negative drug outcome and injury. Many case reports and lawsuits involved individuals who lived alone. It is crucial to have a roommate or spouse present to help identify bizarre behaviors before they become dangerous or life threatening. Consider enlisting a "buddy-sitter" to help monitor your use of any sleep agent, should you continue using these agents.

Dr. Lori Arnold, PharmD

Z-drugs continue to dominate the sleeping pill market with no indication of slowing down. As a consequence, safety issues will keep piling up as people continue to be impacted by unpredictable outcomes that we may never fully understand. In my professional opinion, there is nothing safe about long-term use of sleep agents. Drug warnings are not suggestions—the strictest adherence is mandatory if you continue to take any drug. I assure you the surefire way to ensure your safety is to follow the *undrugged* lifestyle by not taking these drugs in the first place.

CHAPTER 7

Lawsuits and Legal Woes: The "Zolpidem Defense"

> The snowball effect is a process that starts from an initial state of small significance and builds upon itself, becoming larger (graver, more serious), and also perhaps potentially dangerous or disastrous, a "spiral of decline."
> —Wikipedia

The media storm following the very public traffic incident involving Congressman Patrick Kennedy beckoned endless legal opportunity for lawyers. A peak in zolpidem-induced, bizarre behavior reporting prompted a deluge of corresponding personal injury lawsuits against the manufacturers. One witty attorney coined her defendants, "Zolpidem Zombies." Horror stories based on "the pill made me do it" testimonials were told over and over, highlighting extreme situations where individuals in zolpidem trances were arrested for DWI (driving while intoxicated) or even more grisly crimes like murder.

Several lawsuits featured the "zolpidem defense," built on defendants' claims of "I just don't remember." Devastating consequences often dovetail the toxic combination of zolpidem-amnesia, a predisposition for sleepwalking, mixing with alcohol or other drugs. One document of 2011 legal proceedings showed zolpidem was directly implicated in several criminal cases, including seven violent crimes, ten driving-related incidents, and one sex offense. Lawyers argued defendants ingested zolpidem near the time of the incidents in order to reduce criminal liability.[92]

Here are a few actual cases in which people committed criminal acts under the influence of zolpidem. In 2006, after taking zolpidem, a man stabbed his girlfriend twenty-seven times with a pocketknife, claiming he dreamed she was cheating on him. He claimed he suffered complete absence of memory during the entire horrendous act. In 2009, after taking a cocktail of five zolpidem tablets mixed with whiskey and other drugs, a man bludgeoned his roommate to death with a hammer. Two additional cases involved individuals who were both being treated with paroxetine (an SSRI antidepressant known to interact with zolpidem) for depression. After taking 20 mg of zolpidem, a forty-five-year-old man awoke handcuffed in a wheelchair with no recollection that he had stabbed his wife over twenty times, killing her. After taking two or three zolpidem 10 mg tablets, a sixty-two-year-old woman killed her husband by bashing his head several times with a metal pipe and then finished the act by placing a plastic bag over his head.[93] In cases of violent murders, injury, or harm to loved ones, individuals insisted they suffered from total or partial amnesia during the incidents. Though these isolated cases are unnerving and gruesome, mixing the wrong dangerous drug combination in the wrong person can prove deadly.

Zolpidem amnesia has also been implicated in a few disturbing sex crimes and molestation cases. Some experts postulate that "sleep sex" is directly linked to the effect of amnesia enhancing one's lack of inhibition. Unfortunately, sexual predators figured this out and began utilizing zolpidem as a date rape drug.

Is the "zolpidem defense" a valid legal argument? If so, who assumes liability—the manufacturer, the physician, or the patient? We will never know for certain, as each situation presents a host of extenuating circumstances. Today, the "zolpidem defense" is weak due to the public's increased vigilance and the multiple improved explicit warnings and precautions on drug labeling. Prosecutors argue that patients should be very well informed about dangerous interactions and other drug safety risks, as these warnings are extensively documented, highly publicized, and provided by the pharmacy with each drug fill or refill.

CHAPTER 8

Unvitamin Effect: Nutrient Depletions

Nearly all disease can be traced to a nutritional deficiency.
—Dr. Linus Pauling

Studies assessing drug effect on nutrient status are not common practice for most drug companies; therefore, specific nutrient depletions have not been identified with Z-drugs. I offer you this quick disclaimer: Don't automatically assume absence of company data equates to absence of nutrient depletions. Commonalities can be found by analyzing depletions created by other drugs that utilize similar receptor pathways. In this case, GABA-A receptors are acted upon by both anticonvulsants and Z-drugs. Therefore, it is postulated that Z-drug nutrient depletions would be similar to those documented for anticonvulsants. With that in mind, here is a list of potential *unvitamin* effects.[94]

Nutrient Depleted: **Calcium**. Potential Health Problems and Symptoms: brittle bones and osteoporosis, heart and blood pressure irregularities, tooth decay, muscle spasms and twitching
Nutrient Depleted: **Vitamin B1 (thiamine)**. Potential Health Problems and Symptoms: confusion, depression, fatigue, insomnia, irritability, nervousness, memory loss, muscle cramps and weakness
Nutrient Depleted: **Vitamin B7 (biotin)**. Potential Health Problems and Symptoms: anemia, dandruff, depression, dermatitis, hair

loss, hallucinations, lethargy, lowered immunity, numbness and tingling in extremities, muscle pain

Nutrient Depleted: **Vitamin B9 (folic acid)**. Potential Health Problems and Symptoms: anemia, heart disease, depression, fatigue, indigestion, insomnia, irritability, numbness and tingling in extremities, weakness

Nutrient Depleted: **Vitamin B12 (cobalamin)**. Potential Health Problems and Symptoms: anemia, confusion, depression, dizziness, fatigue, hallucinations, insomnia, irritability, memory loss, numbness and tingling in extremities, ringing in ears, stiffness, weakness

Nutrient Depleted: **Vitamin D**. Potential Health Problems and Symptoms: bone loss and osteoporosis, hearing loss, lowered immunity, muscle spasms, and weakness

Nutrient Depleted: **Vitamin K**. Potential Health Problems and Symptoms: bleeding, decreased collagen (makes skin look thinner), kidney stones, osteoporosis, prolonged clotting time, skin bruising

PART II

From Insomnia to Un-somnia: Undrugged Solutions to Naturally Promote Sleep

CHAPTER 9

The Undrugged Method

The best cure for insomnia is to get a lot of sleep.
—W.C. Fields

Undrugged Phase I. Removal of Drug

Every Forty-Year-Old Woman

Dear Dr. *Undrugged*:

I am Every Forty-Year-Old Woman, and I'm sick and tired of being sick and tired. In just a few short years, I have battled a multitude of health issues and have taken dozens of drug treatments and now find my health spiraling out of control. I need help.

As a young child, I caught every cold and flu bug and had constant bouts of bronchitis and recurring sinus infections and ear infections, which subsequently subjected me to an equal number of antibiotic regimens and steroid bursts. As a teen, painful irregular menstruation led to treatment with birth control pills, and hormonal acne was treated with more antibiotics and various topical creams and solutions.

During a routine yearly physical at twenty-four, high cholesterol was discovered, and I was placed on a statin drug, atorvastatin (Lipitor). At twenty-six, while attempting to adjust to a new job and marriage, I suffered from horrible heartburn, which was treated with Tums, ranitidine (Zantac), and eventually esomeprazole (Nexium). At twenty-eight, I developed overwhelming sadness, diagnosed as depression, leading to antidepressant treatment with paroxetine (Paxil).

I continued a downhill spiral in my thirties. At thirty-one, I developed painful and unsightly cystic acne, treated with more antibiotics and eventually the acne-blasting drug, Accutane. At thirty-four, fatigue and hair loss led to a diagnosis of hypothyroidism treated with levothyroxine (Synthroid). At thirty-five, I developed constipation treated with stool softeners and laxatives, and the resulting hemorrhoids were relieved with steroid creams and suppositories. At thirty-six, my inability to fall asleep was diagnosed as insomnia, treatable with nightly zolpidem (Ambien). At thirty-seven, worsening depression added bupropion (Wellbutrin) to my regimen. I feel like a freight train without breaks barreling toward a dead-end cliff; a train wreck is imminent.

I am now forty years old and take twelve routine daily medications. I keep developing additional symptoms and illnesses, for which I am given more medications. I battle food obsessions, uncontrollable cravings, and ravaging hunger. On occasion when blessed with sleep, my dreams are consumed with ooey-gooey brownies oozing with hot fudge and marshmallow crème. A midlife weight gain has found me, and I *feel* like a chunky monkey. My once sassy and svelte figure is now insulated with an extra fifty pounds that bubbles and pops out in the oddest places. I am now a walking smorgasbord with cottage-cheese thighs, a fluffy muffin top, pancake butt, and a back fat donut that spills out under my bra. I have tried every exercise program but always quit because I am just too tired to stick to any program.

After several failed attempts over the years, my husband and I were unable to conceive a child. I currently have no sex drive and am entering menopause; it seems a little early. My husband voices that he constantly feels rejected and threatens to leave, we fight about it, and then I get more depressed. My doctor blames hormones and sent me to a therapist to talk about my problems. I am on an emotional rollercoaster and long to feel good for *just one day*. Is this really all I have to look forward to in my life? Can you please help me?

Yours truly,
Every Forty-Year-Old Woman, aka, Sick and Tired of Being Sick and Tired

Does Every Forty-Year-Old Woman sound like anyone you know? Maybe you can relate personally, or perhaps you see similarities in your wife or maybe even a sister or best friend. Though I created this fictitious scenario, the story closely mirrored my own personal health and illness journey. With just a few minor differences, I was Every Forty-Year-Old Woman; only I peaked at twelve daily medications at the age of thirty-four.

I could have continued on a downward spiral of more medications and more corresponding symptoms had I not broadened my horizons by becoming a more savvy consumer and pharmacist and, subsequently, a fellowship trained, board certified clinician in natural medicine. I was able to successfully taper myself from esomeprazole (Nexium) and all antacid medications and completely heal my acid reflux. All antibiotics I needed to take for acne were stopped, and subsequently all signs of cystic acne disappeared simply by removing food intolerances from my diet. I fixed my gut issues and employed a combined nutraceutical and holistic spiritual approach for my mood imbalance, thus diminishing the need for the antidepressant paroxetine (Paxil). When I learned *how* to sleep, I no longer needed zolpidem (Ambien). I became the first official graduate of the *undrugged* program, and I know it works; I am a living testimonial.

Every Forty-Year-Old Woman demonstrated how each drug taken results in a collection of new subsequent symptoms that stack up over the years. From birth, the moment of exposure to your first vaccine or dose of antibiotic, latent drug effects began to compound like interest in a savings account. Every chemical insult collects in your system and taxes your body's natural detoxification ability. The more medicine you take, the more internal chemical "toxic soup" you create. Most people are unaware that drugs don't stay primarily in the targeted body part they are designed for, thus increasing the likelihood that drug may adversely affect other unrelated bodily systems. This manifests as side effects, under the guise of new symptoms, which mask as completely new diseases. Rather than investigating a current medication's cascade of side effects, a new drug is often added instead, and thus continues an unending cycle of overdrugging. Years of my own clinical experience have helped uncover trends and commonalities, with disturbingly predictable adverse outcomes from regular medication use, even when used exactly as prescribed by doctors. Knowing this, why would you continue on this vicious cycle? Why would you *not* want to become *undrugged*?

Now that you know better, you *should* do better. It is crystal clear that the insomnia solution isn't just a tiny pill away, and the last few chapters should have solidified this point. I held nothing back when I provided an up-to-date, accurate, raw, and uncut Z-drug assessment with all pharma fluff and smoking screens removed.

Long-term sleeping pill use leads to a tsunami of horrible and devastating consequences. You may think you can learn to live with some bothersome side effects; however, more serious reactions could potentially lead to deadly repercussions. As a prime example, I was fortunate to have my own zolpidem stupor end with a temporary and annoying bloated belly and food coma, rather than suffering a careless stumble that catapulted me over the balcony, potentially ending in serious injury or death. Armed with an abundance of valuable Z-drug knowledge, you should now look forward to embarking on your own drug-free *undrugged* healing journey, using effective alternative means to conquer your sleep woes. At this time, you deserve props, and I would like to personally congratulate you, as you are now more informed about Z-drugs than most physicians, pharmacists, and other health care providers.

With certainty, a codependent sleeping pill relationship has no future; it's a dead-end, unhealthy attachment that must cease. Free yourself by breaking up with your sleeping drug. To begin *Undrugged* Phase I, Removal of Drug, I recommend collaboration with a healthcare provider before stopping any drug therapy. If your provider doesn't support discontinuing your sleep drug, seek another opinion from an integrative physician or naturopath who will prioritize identifying the root cause of your sleep issue in order to safely taper and stop drug treatment. Extra emphasis is placed on "taper," as quitting sleep agents "cold turkey" after continuous use can be uncomfortable and stressful after your body is physically and mentally dependent on the drug. When I tapered myself off of zolpidem, I began by cutting the dose by half for one week. After one week, I reduced the dose further to a quarter of the original dose for one week. After two weeks, I stopped the zolpidem and only used it sparingly as needed. Recall, discontinuation of Z-drugs after prolonged use will lead to withdrawal rebound insomnia, which is a temporary worsening of sleeplessness. To lessen the severity of your symptoms, ensuring a more successful outcome, I highly stress adhering to a *gradual taper*, similar to the tapering regimen I employed on myself, lasting a few days to weeks, augmented with the implementation of other insomnia solutions found throughout Part II. You may find some of the nutraceutical products I suggest will help bridge your taper and reduce the severity of the rebound insomnia. Rather than enveloping yourself in a drug haze, the *undrugged* approach shifts focus to the root cause of your sleep-related issue. You may be pleasantly surprised how quickly you could be enjoying restoration of normal sleep patterns and freedom from the barrage of unpleasant side effects.

My goal is to inspire the adoption of an *undrugged* philosophy. I have already noted an encouraging shift in mainstream medicine where more physicians are embracing nondrug options as effective insomnia treatments. In fact, literature recommends cognitive behavioral therapy (CBT) as first-line insomnia treatment, before progressing to sleeping pill use. CBT is no small undertaking for the patient or the provider—it takes concerted effort in order to work. Administering CBT requires a five-hour time commitment for four to six weeks, followed by monthly maintenance.[95] Sessions utilize psychology to target misconceptions about sleep, insomnia, and perceived daytime consequences. In addition, patients are also provided stimulus control, sleep restriction therapy, relaxation training, and education. Studies showed CBT to be equally as effective as sleeping pills. However, a mere 1 percent of chronic insomniacs actually practice this technique. A major CBT downfall is lack of appropriate training for health care professionals, along with time and resource limitations. As a result, a majority of doctors opt for prescribing an easy pill fix when faced with a sleep-distressed patient.[96] Some patients may require an intense level of intervention with close medical oversight, like CBT. For many, however, simply utilizing this book and the tools provided may prove more beneficial. The *undrugged* method worked for me, and it can work for you.

Dr. Lori Arnold, PharmD

Undrugged **Personal Empowerment**

To successfully complete Phase I, and even before you attempt to remove any drug from your regimen, you have to overcome any limiting beliefs you may have about yourself.

Personally, I firmly adhere to this philosophy—I've been there and done that. As a professional, I deem it necessary for you to adopt a winning belief system as well. A spirited *undrugged* pep talk is warranted and will provide an extra dose of personal empowerment.

You don't need that stinkin' sleeping pill, so dump the drug. Never let anybody, including your doctor, tell you that you can't do this. Motivational speaker Les Brown hit the mark when he said, "People who can't see it for themselves can't see it for you!" These are prolific words of motivation. If you have established a clear goal to get *undrugged*, do your best to surround yourself with those who believe in you and your mission. Detoxing from prescription drug therapy may seem like a foreign concept to many people. They may not get it, may not understand it. And because they are fearful of stepping outside their own comfort zone, they may assume it won't work for you. That is a big lie, and it simply is not true. Be unafraid of stepping into the unknown. In one of my favorite songs, "Standing Outside the Fire," country music artist Garth Brooks says, "You've got to be tough when consumed by desire, 'cause it's not enough just to stand outside the fire." When you are on the verge of the biggest healing breakthrough of your life, you may be hit with great opposition. Opposition is like a parasite; it is the "enemy," and it can strike you full force in the form of naysayers who are friends, family, or even your medical professionals. The most impactful motivational speeches I ever heard were from those who told me I could not do it. Don't ever let them tell you that can't do it. Prove them wrong. Show the naysayers you can achieve anything you commit to. You need discipline—make yourself accountable to yourself. Decide, commit, act, and repeat. In your heart, if you believe you can reach this goal, you have planted a seed, and this victory is meant for you. Keep pursuing it. Be a fierce lion, not a sheep. Take control of the situation and stand firmly by your decision to heal any health issue. In the Bible, Jesus said, "Be not afraid." I encourage you to cast fear aside, along with all seeds of doubt, and instead focus on nourishing a positive mind-set.

If you want to end the codependent relationship with your sleeping drug badly enough, just do it. Remember, the solution can only be found *within you,* and you are most capable of getting the job done. Tap into your power of perseverance and confidence and continuously nourish an unwavering belief in your own ability to eliminate sleeping drug dependence. Be audacious—be bold, daring, recklessly brave, and fearless—and you will be victorious.

TEDWomen recently featured the dynamo Maysoon Zayid. She is an actress, comedian, and activist who is a self-proclaimed "Palestinian Muslim virgin with cerebral palsy from New Jersey." Despite naysayers, she has overcome physical disability and has reached success in many areas of her life. Her father, who constantly encouraged her to defy the odds, instilled a winning belief system in his young daughter. Your personal healing mission can be strengthened by Maysoon's personal mantra, "If I can can, you can can!" If she can defy the odds, so "can can" you.

"The first time I tried to stop taking zolpidem, I failed. The second time I tried to stop taking zolpidem, I failed. Failure made me try harder and instilled a stronger desire to overcome this seemingly unreachable goal. The third time I tapered my zolpidem, I succeeded—for the long term."

—Dr. Lori Arnold

Business success coach Denis Waitley teaches seminars on mental toughness, or the philosophy of creating a winning mind-set. This mind-set is designed to help you overcome challenges in life. It is closely related to my *undrugged* process that employs the body's natural ability to heal from within. While developing mental toughness, we will encounter surprises along the way, Waitley assures, surprises that most likely will manifest as negative experiences. Many view negative experiences as failures. For instance, utilizing a slow taper to remove a sleeping drug will cause physical consequences, like rebound insomnia. This does not constitute a treatment failure; rather, it is part of your healing journey that must be overcome. The key to success with the *undrugged* process will be how you deal with any negative physical symptoms; are you going to make a mountain out of a molehill, or will you keep a molehill a molehill? Physical symptoms for a few days are merely a temporary inconvenience, or a stumbling stone along the way. If at first you do not succeed at tapering the drug, try again. Do not give up. I know all too well from all of my *undrugged* processes, failure was merely an event; failure did not dictate my future success. The first time I tried to stop taking zolpidem, I failed. The second time I tried to stop taking zolpidem, I failed. The first time you try to taper off of your sleeping pill, you may fail. Get back up and try again. Failure made me try harder, and instilled a stronger desire to overcome this seemingly unreachable goal. The third time I tapered my zolpidem, I succeeded—for the long term. Waitley says, "Failure is the fertilizer of success. Failure stinks, it smells. Fertilize life with your mistakes; don't wallow in it or lie in it. Learn from it and move on." Failure is a detour; mind-set is the compass that resets your course. Winnie the Pooh said it best: "There is something you must always remember. You are braver than you believe, stronger than you seem, and smarter than you think."

> "If I can can, you can can!"
> —Maysoon Zayid, actress, comedian, activist

Undrugged Phase II. Reverse and Recover: Learning to Heal

> If your goal is to achieve optimal health, one essential nonnegotiable requirement is sleep—lack of sleep causes illness and promotes chronic disease.
> —Dr. Lori Arnold

Like an internal tattoo, Z-drugs leave a lasting impression on your body, especially if used long-term. In almost all cases, exposure to any Z-drug insult should be followed by recovery, allowing adequate time to repair damaging side effects and restore natural biorhythms. Like hitting a computer's reset button, your neurotransmitters are hardwired to instinctively know exactly what to do. Sleep is a primal need, like eating. You are the technician responsible for providing your body with the means to do so. Removing zolpidem from my sleep routine was not an easy undertaking. I found my biggest hurdle was overcoming mind games. After an extended period of dependence on zolpidem to induce sleep, I was thoroughly convinced that I would never be able to achieve a decent night of sleep unless I took a pill. I let fear lead my actions and resisted shifting my thoughts to a faith-based mind-set. Once I committed to trusting in my own ability to successfully eradicate this bad habit, I let go of limiting beliefs and willed my thoughts to remain focused and determined; I let faith lead the way. Your body is intelligent and will follow where your mind leads it; you just need to direct your cells to respond to positive and encouraging affirmations. Lead your body into recovery and be gentle and kind to yourself when choosing your methodology. Each individual will heal at his or her own pace, so be patient with the process and don't give up. I never said it would be easy, but I guarantee it will be worth it.

A firm commitment to eradicate your insomnia without drugs requires an arsenal of resources to assure your success. *Undrugged Sleep* supplies you with a toolbox of options to help you establish healthier, more supportive habits to achieve gratifying sleep. You will rewire your learned response of reaching for a sleeping pill "Band-Aid," thereby redirecting your internal circuitry with a desire to find and fix the root cause of the underlying sleep malfunction. Typically, insomnia is a collection of bad habits that continuously build on each other until it eventually becomes unmanageable. Reflect and ask yourself, how are my sleep habits, good or bad? Honestly assessing your personal regimen can unveil crucial clues that lead to the discovery of your sleep wreckers.

During *Undrugged* Phase II, Reverse and Recover, I urge you to analyze your habits—to identify personal sleep-sabotaging factors through a series of relatable scenarios. Once you have pinpointed specific "sleep thieves," you can begin tweaking your routine using natural treatments. *Undrugged* Phase II is further broken down into the following segments—readjust, replenish and restore, and refresh. First, you will *readjust* your habits to improve sleep hygiene. Next, you will *replenish and restore* potential depletions with sleepy-time supplements and herbs. And finally, you will *refresh* your nutrition by adding relaxing, sleep-promoting foods and avoiding sleep-stealing

Dr. Lori Arnold, PharmD

foods. There is no particular order in which you should enact these steps, and you can mix and match as many of these tips as needed. Once you have created your own effective personal sleepy-time blend, you will be on your way to more rejuvenating and restorative sleep.

CHAPTER 10

Readjust: Adopt Better Sleep Habits

A good laugh and a long sleep are the best cures in the doctor's book.
—Irish Proverb

After personally suffering from insomnia for extended periods of time, I realized that I'd been missing out on sleep's crucial health benefits. For the average individual, seven to nine hours of rejuvenating sleep is needed every night to reap the rewards of increased energy, creativity, and self-esteem; enhanced problem solving and cognition; and increased overall happiness. Some people can function perfectly with less sleep than that, but I am not one of the lucky ones. I need eight solid hours to feel refreshed. Again, sleep is a *priority*, not a luxury. Therefore, wisely organize your daily schedule to allow your body the rest it requires and desires. Denying adequate downtime can prime your body for sluggish immunity with more coughs, colds, and infections; undesirable stomach woes; overwhelming mental overload; and, eventually, physical and emotional burnout. If I suffer from a few days of unproductive sleep, I immediately can identify the ensuing symptoms. I typically experience nausea and unsettled digestion or out-of-whack, unhealthy food cravings; lethargy, low exercise tolerance, and weakness that makes me more prone to injury in the gym; unsightly, dark circles under my eyes; muscle aches and pains; low motivation, mood swings with a tendency toward sadness or irritability, and an allover feeling of unease and stress. How does lack of sleep manifest physically or mentally for you?

Resorting to pill popping for sleep is an act of desperation—a byproduct of the ingrained, stuck thought process that says, "I've tried *everything*, and it hasn't worked." Have you really tried everything?

Let it be said, "You don't know what you don't know." Therefore, if no one offered you other options, you probably assumed a pill was your only solution. Did any of your physicians ask about your "sleep hygiene" and initiate a discussion about your habits before scribbling a script? Most likely, that can of worms couldn't be opened in the rushed five minutes he spent with you. Sleep hygiene is not a method to combat body odor. Rather, it is a collection of nightly routines you and I practice before going to bed. Regardless, forced chemical induction of sleep begs for reassessment of your current situation. I'd like to give you a little food for thought in the next section by targeting areas you may need to overhaul in order to successfully *readjust* your sleep hygiene.

Rest and Digest: Mindful Eating

Simply, poor eating habits sabotage sleep.

Are late night dinners your forte? Do you frequently find yourself at social gatherings enjoying sumptuous, heavy evening feasts, overindulging on Texas-sized steaks, loaded baked potatoes, and decadent chocolate desserts—all washed down with a heavy-handed pour of Merlot wine? I sincerely hope you answered no if you are struggling with sleep issues. There are always invitations to evening celebrations where food is the main attraction, and I am confident that, if you are like me, you will grant yourself a "hall pass," allowing a time or two of late-night overeating. Beware; a few moments of blissful food ecstasy may be short-lived, backfiring with hours of excruciating acid reflux, bloating, belching, gas, and an angry colon. Resist the "urge to purge" the burn with an antacid—this was self-inflicted suffering.

If you consume a heavy dinner, you shift digestion into overdrive, taxing your gut for hours. This is a counterproductive response—redirecting energy resources to meal breakdown, not sleep. Adding insult to injury, super-sized protein portions at nighttime may be overstimulating for some, providing an ill-timed energy boost and a delayed blood sugar response. You can ease nighttime digestion workload by going meatless for evening meals or by consuming smaller protein portions of fish or poultry. A bulk of your meal should also contain easily digestible vegetables and healthy grains, like quinoa or brown rice pasta, and always go easy or eliminate spicy and fatty foods.

Just say, "No!" to nightly decadent desserts and sweet, chocolaty treats. Most desserts contain both refined sugars and caffeine, which create erratic blood sugar fluctuations and undesirable stimulation. Carefully monitor caffeine content in all food and drink, and pass when offered an after-dinner espresso or cup of English tea. Most people tend to overlook the caffeine found in most black, white, and green herbal teas, and the especially high caffeine content found in matcha green tea. To avoid excessive evening stimulation, I encourage you to cease caffeine consumption at lunchtime, as the effects can last *up to eight hours*, or even longer in more sensitive individuals.[97]

Although "wine and dine" go hand in hand, resist that *assumed* relaxing glass of wine or nightcap. We've been duped by an unfortunate misconception that alcohol enhances sleep. One sensible cocktail, not a jumbo, eight-ounce wine pour or fishbowl margarita may provide a soothing and satisfying experience. However, I know firsthand, when enjoying a nightcap, it can become easy to justify another one, two, or even more. Alcohol is a known sleep disruptor, and studies have confirmed that the body's restorative functions are hindered after a single alcoholic beverage, with further intensification of the detrimental effects with each additional libation.[98]

What should I do? It is simple—adhere to centuries of wisdom and "eat like a pauper" at dinner, making it the smallest meal of the day. Maintain a strict regimen of reserving evenings for resting and digesting. The basic rule of thumb is to finish eating at least two to three hours prior to bedtime, allowing adequate digestion before lying down. Additional health benefits, including weight loss, can be gained by allowing a minimum of ten to twelve hours' fast between dinner and breakfast. For a more detailed discussion on sleep nutrition and appropriate eating habits, refer to chapter 13, "Refresh: Healing with Food."

Undrugged Tidbit: Prevent Nighttime Heartburn

To avoid indigestion and the temptation to reach for a nightly antacid, finish eating at least two to three hours prior to bedtime and do not lay down immediately after eating dinner.

Book an Appointment and Set the Mood

Book a nightly sleep appointment on an established schedule. Set an official sleep time and do your best to go to bed and wake up at the same time every day. Like prepping for a marathon, you need to be consistent and mindful of your routine. Dedicated athletes do not skip training sessions; therefore, in order to successfully overcome insomnia, you will need to be faithful to your sleep time slot while you are conditioning new behaviors. It may be tempting to justify shorting yourself a couple minutes here and there, but don't do it. Minutes will eventually become more minutes, turning into hours, which will ultimately decondition you and annihilate your efforts. Program a "lights off" habit by choosing your ideal bedtime based on when you feel sleepiest. Adjusting to a new routine takes time. Therefore, if you are still awake after twenty minutes of lying in bed with the lights off, get up and do something relaxing for a few minutes. Stressing and obsessing about sleep only prolongs your agony and makes you more anxious and frustrated. If you remain adherent to a scheduled sleep-wake pattern, you will successfully reset your internal circadian biorhythm and eventually wake up automatically without the assistance of an alarm clock. Wouldn't you love to avoid an annoying morning wake-up call?

This may sound familiar: "I have way too much to get done before I can go to bed." Life in the fast lane, coupled with a need to succeed, may have you frazzled at the end of the day, as you desperately struggle to accomplish as much as possible before admitting defeat with sleep. Say I if you are guilty of engaging in late-night email-a-thons or if you get completely engrossed in useless Facebook or Instagram scroll-a-thons. Say I if you fall into a hypnotic time warp while lying in bed watching silly "a cucumber freaked out my cat"

YouTube videos on your smartphone. Newsflash: As you are mindlessly preoccupying yourself with these time-wasting activities, funds are draining out of your precious sleep bank. You become oblivious that your overstimulating, media-induced trance is forcing an excitatory state that is keeping your brain aroused, not tired. Unfortunately, a selfie-obsessed society has trained us to be socially connected twenty-four hours a day. As a result, electronics have become our new bedmates, allowing us to indulge in internet multitasking while watching television and Snapchatting with our friends—all at the same time. Even when spouses are in bed together, many become too distracted to engage in meaningful conversation or intimacy. What happened to the days of reading books or snuggling in bed? If you value sleep, it's time to cut the cord, disable the Wi-Fi, and reboot your routine by shutting down all gizmos and "techy tools" an hour or more prior to bedtime. Keep your bedroom device-free; this includes nixing the television.

Be aware that bright lights at night are too stimulating—mood lighting is not just for lovers. Dim or shut off lights at least one to two hours prior to going to bed. Artificial and ambient electronic lighting, including computers, phones, and televisions, lowers hormonal production of your "sleep hormone," melatonin, which regulates sleep-wake cycles and aids in the production of your "happy hormone," serotonin. Because your body produces peak levels of melatonin between 10:00 p.m. and 2:00 a.m., it is crucial to be *sleeping* in a dark room during those hours. For optimal hormonal function, train your body to support a bedtime prior to 10:00 p.m.

You've dimmed the lights and broken your device-in-bed habit. What other modifiable factors should you consider? Like Goldilocks and the Three Bears, your bedroom should be *not too hot and not too cold*—even that clever, pigtailed little girl knew the temperature had to be *just right*. You may notice that you sleep better with the windows open, a fan turned on, or even while camping under the stars. My best sleep was found on chilly North Dakota winter nights under layers of down-filled comforters with handmade afghans pulled over my ears. Cooler climates force you to roll into a blanket burrito and get "snug as a bug in a rug." A slight drop in core body temperature helps induce sleep. To further enhance your chances for sleep success, make sure to set your bedroom thermostat between sixty-five and seventy-two degrees.

Dr. Lori Arnold, PharmD

The temperature is set; the lights are turned down low. Now what? Bustling activity rivaling Grand Central Station belongs in New York City, not in your bedroom. Reserve your bedroom as your private sanctuary restricted to sleep and sex. Unclutter your room, allowing you to only associate it with restful time. That may mean you will have to remove the dust-collecting stationary bike or treadmill you've kept wedged in the corner for use as a modified clothesline. Work projects can be a tremendous source of stress and belong in your office, not in your bedroom. Beds are for sleeping, not eating. Therefore, all food belongs in the kitchen, not in bed. And as long as we are on the subject of *what not to bring to bed*, be aware that you may be forfeiting precious sleep by allowing children and pets to sleep with you. What parent hasn't been kicked in the shin or smacked in the face by a jumpy child vividly dreaming? Restless children wake up frequently, meaning you will too. As a fellow fur baby lover, I do understand the desire to snuggle fur babies in bed. However, much like children, pets are fidgety and prone to nighttime wanderings, and they can also trigger hay fever symptoms by introducing dander and environmental allergens to your bed.

I've given you a few ideas on how to prime your sleep environment. Now, I need to acclimate you to a "wind down" pattern at least two to three hours before bedtime. If your ideal relaxing evening involves television, be discerning with the content of your programming. If you are like my older sister, you may love a chilling thriller or horror flick that gives you goose bumps, makes your hair stand on end, raises your heart rate, and makes it hard to breathe. You may even crave that nail-biting adrenaline rush; unfortunately, *overstimulation* from movies and television programs can provoke anxiety, increase stress hormones, and contribute to restless sleep. Laugh if you will. I sometimes get anxious watching the Food Network's program *Chopped*. For those unfamiliar with this cooking contest craze, four skilled chefs are thrown into a kitchen and tasked with creating a there-course meal out of wacky and ridiculous basket ingredients, like hundred-year-old egg, lamb fries, or gummy bears—under an insane time limit pressure. Though not quite as intense as *Silence of the Lambs, Saw,* or *Jaws*, it may be nerve-racking for some.

Apply the same rule if you prefer unwinding with a good book. Wisely choose content and opt for semiboring or funny material. Your new objective is to avoid overactivating your brain. Unwise selections include complex textbooks like quantum physics, suspenseful Sidney Sheldon or Dan Brown page-turning mysteries, or grisly Stephen King spine-chillers like *Pet Cemetery*. Better choices I would suggest may include inspirational or devotional books, like the Bible or anything written by Louise Hay or Wayne Dyer, along with prayer, meditation, positive affirmations, and mantras. Essentially, read the "good book," but don't read a book that is *too good*—you will further fuel your insomnia by creating a book hangover, which is next-day fatigue induced by staying up too late reading a book you can't put down. I must admit, I am guilty of this and am no stranger to book hangovers.

Music is medicine and is a wonderfully effective sleep treatment that syncs your body to healthy, natural rhythms.[99] Research has even shown thirty minutes of music therapy can produce similar effects to 10 mg of the popular antianxiety agent, diazepam (Valium).[100] You can mellow out and de-stress with music or soothing nature sounds from a white noise sound machine. Here is the caveat, once more; wise song selection is paramount for the appropriate body response. Slow and subdued music, like Bach and Deuter, lowers heart rate and slows breathing, while chaotic, fast-paced music, like Green Day or Pitbull, quickens heart rate and is energizing. Select instrumental music, devoid of irritating noises that may wake you, like crashing cymbals or eerie noises like whining orcas, with a beat that matches your normal pulse. Native American and other ethnic instrumental pieces from India, Ireland, Tibet, and Japan have very soothing selections.

Certain music compositions are specifically designed to aid in healing like ambient or New Age, utilizing vibrational energy of tuning forks, gongs, singing crystal bowls, and nondistracting drumming. Solfeggio is a scientific school of music that repairs disease at a cellular level using healing frequencies. Sleep and deep relaxation are often associated with solfeggio at frequencies of 528 hertz (Hz) and 432 Hz, selections of which you can easily download to your smartphone. My favorite solfeggio composition is a seven-CD set you can easily purchase on Amazon.com or MichaelTyrrell.com called *Wholetones*, by Michael Tyrrell. *Wholetones* was created to promote positive, healthy change. I specifically enjoy a 417 Hz solfeggio called *Desert Sojourn*, with frequencies that are touted to help break negative cycles such as procrastination, self-medication, and eating junk food and that may help if you suffer from sluggishness and lethargy. My other favorite is a 528 Hz piece called *Transformation*, said to help restore broken DNA, the source of disease. Michael Tyrrell offers another three-CD set, also available in a downloadable version for your phone or computer called *Wholetones: Life, Love and Lullabies.* This set was created specifically to promote healthy, peaceful, and restorative sleep. You will find another 528 Hz selection in this set called "All Through the Night," a lullaby from Wales.

    If you do not want to purchase a CD set, you can also utilize internet radio services, like Pandora, to access beneficial sleep-promoting stations like Sounds of Nature, Relaxation and Spa, and Yoga. If you make appropriate selections, you will be lulled to sleep with lapping ocean waves, humming woodwinds, or reverberations from calming vibrational tones. As a bonus, many of these programs have sleep timers you can set on your smartphone to shut off automatically at designated times. To help myself sleep, I set my Pandora to the Yoga station and my phone timer to thirty minutes. I lay on my back, arms to my sides, palms facing upward. I utilize deep breathing and focus on clearing my mind in order to pray, express gratitude for my blessings, or quietly reflect on my healing mantras and affirmations. I encourage you to try this technique.

    I have one last crucial piece of advice; ditch old-school digital alarm clocks that reside on your nightstand. You may not realize that sleep is hindered by the glow of the clock's ambient light combined with the stress-inducing urge to obsessively clock watch. Opt for using the alarm function on your cell phone, with the ringer switched off or the emergency mode turned on, and be sure to flip the phone over to avoid illuminating the room with the screen's glow. For your personal safety and to prevent unneeded electromagnetic frequency exposure (EMF), always store cell phones away from the bed and disable the Wi-Fi mode. Cell phone radiation has been shown to increase alertness by activating brain stress systems, thus hindering the ability to fall asleep and reach deeper sleep stages.

Schedule a Test Rest to Sleep on a Cloud

> For vigor and zest get unbroken rest. The secret of glowing health and radiant beauty often lies in the hours of revitalizing rest you get from your night's sleep.
>
> —1940s Sealy mattress ad

It sounds so enticing; you may even be tempted to splurge on a plush pillow top right now. Quality rest is directly linked to the condition of your sleep surface. Your decrepit mattress or crusty old pillow could actually be your sneaky sleep thief. Perform a mattress assessment. Does your sleep surface resemble a motocross racetrack, full of dips, grooves, lumps, and bumps? Do you have to frequently flip and rotate your mattress to locate that one "sweet spot" that won't leave you with a stiff neck, sore back, or achy hips or aggravate your sciatica? I'll get right to the point: When was the last time you replaced your mattress? Oddly enough, mattresses are not high on most people's priority list of necessities needing replacement. It is not uncommon for many to sleep on the same uncomfortable, shoddy mattress for fifteen, twenty, or even thirty years. Much like a safety blanket, some people develop "mattress separation anxiety," making it too difficult to let go. Lumpy, broken-down mattresses belong in a landfill, not in your bedroom.

If this sounds all too familiar to you, schedule a "test rest" in a mattress showroom. Treat the experience like buying a car; most of you wouldn't purchase a car without a test drive, so don't risk buying a mattress without a test rest. According to the National Sleep Foundation, a good mattress should last nine to ten years; however, if you notice you are not sleeping well, you should be replace it after five to seven years. If you are still apprehensive about the $1,000 to $2,000 purchase due to the affordability of this high-ticket item, I have convincing justification that will help you overcome this excuse. Most people spend an average of $30,000 on a new car; my newest Mazda purchase was $34,000. Most cars are driven an average of one to two hours daily, which equals roughly 5 percent of each day. If you adhere to expert recommendations of achieving eight hours of sleep each night, that would be the equivalent of approximately 33 percent of a twenty-four-hour day spent in bed, or 2,900 hours a year. Compare that to the average time spent in a car yearly, which equates to roughly 730 hours a year (unless, of course, your job includes excessive business travel), and you clearly see why a mattress expenditure is warranted. Bite the bullet and invest in a high-quality mattress.

After upgrading your sleep surface, make a pillow overhaul. Your relationship with your pillow can be funny; you may get territorial with it and fight bedroom battles over it. Most people know it takes a good six months to break in a new one. The standard for most people is to have one primary pillow; however, some prefer creating a pillow nest that can be smashed, bent, and contorted until a comfortable head crater is formed. I have pillow attachment syndrome and know exactly which pillow is mine because it is squished just right and fits perfectly with the shape of my noggin. I also have a spare pillow kept for the sole purpose of preventing my knees from rubbing when I sleep on my side. Jesting aside, when was the last time you replaced your pillow? Experts recommend replacing pillows at least once a year. I don't want to gross you out too much, but be aware that your mangled, sweaty pillow is a cesspool of hair and body oil secretions trapped in the fabric and stuffing. Conditions become favorable for breeding bacteria, putrid odors, and dust mites (yes, bugs), thus contributing to increased allergies and asthma-type symptoms. I urge you to adopt a good habit of replacing pillows yearly at the same time you change batteries in your smoke detectors.

De-Stress: Count Blessings Not Sheep and Learn to Breathe Right

> The curing of the part should not be attempted without treatment of the whole. No attempt should be made to cure the body without the soul and if the head and the body are to be healthy, you must begin by curing the mind ... For this is the great error of our day in the treatment of the human body, that physicians first separate the soul from the body.
> —Plato, third century BC

Stress is a thief in the night, the stealer of dreams, the boogeyman lurking in your head. It throws your monkey mind onto a hamster wheel, keeping you awake and preventing you from reaching a state of calm and peace. After removing all triggers like food, environment, technology, and sleep surface sabotages, you *must* focus on mastering stress reduction. This is a *must* requirement, not a *should* suggestion. Famous business guru Tony Robbins has said, "Don't *should* all over yourself!" *Should* is not making a solid commitment to yourself and merely implies that you are making a suggestion to yourself that you may or may not need to implement into your routine. *Must*, on the other hand, is a firm commitment and promise to yourself that explicitly stresses the importance of removing all excuses, pushing you to make the necessary changes you are required to complete in order to de-stress your sleep routine. Once you tenaciously dedicate yourself to the goal of stress reduction, you will reap health benefits that extend far beyond just sleep improvement.

Undrugging requires you to commit to as many sleep-promoting healing strategies as possible. Incorporating these changes into your routine is not meant to add more stress; rather, these modifications should enhance many aspects of your life. Journaling, deep breathing, meditation, Reiki, and massage are just a few effective sleepiness techniques, as well as enjoying a comforting mug of herbal tea, a warm bath with soothing sea salts and essential oils, calming and cleansing music (like solfeggio), or reading an appropriately selected book. List all activities that normally make you sleepy and try to integrate as many of these relaxing tasks into your evenings as possible. You *must* do what works for you.

I deal with the "hamster wheel" effect by setting my brain's internal taskmaster to paper, and I encourage you to do the same. Basically, wipe your slate clean and get organized every night. Before bed, establish a nightly ritual of journaling your thoughts in a notebook. Reserve a few moments each night to formulate a list of next-day goals, plotting out a generalized to-do list. Target only three to five high-priority tasks, resisting the urge to bog yourself down with a list of petty errands and duties that will only make your day appear more daunting and overwhelming. A directed laser focus will help you avoid the brain-taxing ruminating and mental list making that keeps your monkey mind active and alert. Keep it simple, write it down, and set it aside

---

Count blessings, not sheep, for improved sleep.
—Dr. Lori Arnold

To further reduce stress and anxiety, as well as lower blood pressure, you *must* learn *how to breathe*—the right way. Instead of counting sheep to sleep, *count your blessings* and slow your breathing. Become more aware of each breath, focusing intently on each

Dr. Lori Arnold, PharmD

inhalation and exhalation. By doing so, you will distract your mind from stressful thoughts, clear your mind, restore calm and peace, release body tension, and maintain a focus on the present moment. I encourage you to take a few moments now, as you read this, to feel the sensation of slow, deep, and thoughtful breathing, noticing how an unconscious, automatic function can be consciously controlled. I frequently practice another effective technique called "deep belly breathing," as it has been shown to slow heart rate and interrupt overproduction of the stress hormone cortisol. This method is very simple and will only cost you a few moments of time. Lie in bed with your eyes closed. Like inflating a balloon, inhale deeply through your nose concentrating on filling your lungs and belly with air. Hold each breath for a five or more count, and then slowly exhale until you have let all the air out of your balloon. Repeat several times until you feel relaxed or fall asleep. Thoughtful breathing is an adaptive habit that can be utilized any time you encounter stressful situations, day or night. I find, when I intentionally slow my breathing for a few moments, I am more capable of successfully handling stressful situations like traffic in Los Angeles or a harried and fast-paced day in a busy retail pharmacy.

Undrugged Tidbit: Better Breathing for Asthmatics

Hey asthmatics! Resist the urge to reach for your rescue inhaler if your lungs feel a bit tight. Instead, slow episodes of labored breathing back to normal using deep belly breathing to relax and open lungs.

After mastering the art of thoughtful breathing, you can graduate to meditation. Saint Francis De Sales said, "Where there is peace and meditation, there is neither anxiety nor doubt." Meditation, combined with deep breathing, creates a tranquil state of mind that directs attention to thoughts, feelings, and sensations. When used for insomnia, meditation helps improve coping skills, and reduces stress, fear, worry, anxiety, pain perception, and depressive feelings.[101] From your head to your feet, meditation incorporates full-body relaxation, releasing tension and stiffness and making your body floppy like a wet noodle and flow like Jell-O. If you are still experiencing distracting thoughts, quickly redirect your focus to relaxation. Once centered, slow your breathing until you are overcome with sleep. Like deep breathing, meditation can be used throughout the day as needed.

High-strung personalities or relaxation novices, who have not mastered the art of being still, may require additional interventions and resources to aid with mind calming. One such often-overlooked stress-reducing technique is a form of energy healing called Reiki. For this technique to work, you are asked to keep an open heart and mind, resisting the urge to overthink or overanalyze the process. Though a spiritual practice, Reiki is not a religion, cult, or special belief system. It originated as a healing practice used by Tibetan Buddhists to transfer energy from practitioner to client. A typical session lasts thirty to ninety minutes, often does not involve direct touch, does not use needles or special tools, does not hurt, and only requires that you relax, free of judgment. This practice is becoming more mainstream in the medical field and is used in tandem with essential oils and incense in hospitals and other health care settings.

I began my Reiki practice three years ago with the help of my Reiki master, Richard. I was suffering from a severe case of toxic mold poisoning, which causes a "hot brain" that manifests as extreme bouts of anger, aggression, and anxiety. Any form of negativity and aggression, not necessarily as a result of toxic mold poisoning, can course through your body like black, sluggish tar. Embracing destructive emotions encourages disease and illness, while hindering the healing process. Through my Reiki practice, with the devoted guidance of my skilled practitioner, I was able to purge negative energy and the toxic energetic tar from my body and redirect my internal energy to a healing mind-set with encouraging affirmations and prayers. I still utilize Reiki frequently when I feel an energetic disconnect from my true self and have further advanced my practice to include helping others expel energetic toxicities so they can reach a peaceful state in mind, body, and soul. When used for insomnia treatment, Reiki aids in deep relaxation; helps reduce stress, tension, and anxiety; and decreases anger and agitation.[1021] If done appropriately, in tandem with other *undrugged* solutions, Reiki can be an effective adjunct stress reduction method and a safe way to holistically tackle insomnia—no drugs required.

Dr. Lori Arnold, PharmD

A "Good Tired": Exercise Early

Exercise helps induce a sleepy state and improves overall sleep quality by boosting a "good tired" at night. As a bonus, exercise also enhances your mood and reduces stress levels by stimulating crucial relaxation brain chemicals, like serotonin, dopamine, and norepinephrine.[103] Research showed fifty to seventy-six-year-old insomniacs who engaged in low-impact aerobics or walked briskly thirty minutes daily, four days a week, fell asleep more quickly and slept better for longer periods with fewer awakenings.[104] For some, exercise is the equivalent of a sleeping pill—making it a winning *undrugged*-approved drug substitution. Make exercise a daily requirement, allocating thirty to sixty minutes every day, no excuses; after all, this is only 4 percent of your entire day. Timing is crucial; therefore, in order to promote satisfying sleep, do not exercise *vigorously* two to three hours prior to bedtime. Reserve that time slot for relaxing and slowing down your body, not running a 5K or participating in a "spin to win" cycling class. You may enjoy a leisurely evening walk on the beach to enjoy fresh ocean air, as this does not constitute *vigorous* exercise.

No sleep discussion would be complete without mentioning yoga, a practice that embodies all good sleep-promoting habits like stretching, deep breathing, and meditation.[105] Thousands of studies validate the physical and mental benefits of yoga, showing only three yoga sessions a week can boost GABA levels, thus improving mood and decreasing anxiety.[106] Z-drugs work through GABA receptors. Therefore, it makes perfect sense for me to recommend replacing Z-drugs with yoga. One simple rule, if you practice yoga in the evening, make sure it is the right kind of *gentle* yoga, not vigorous *vinyasa*, *ashtanga*, or *bikram* yoga, which can be energizing. Instead choose *yin* or *restorative* yoga practices that incorporate relaxing poses like tree, forward fold, down dog, cat and cow, child, happy baby, reclined butterfly, and corpse (savasana). "Lying like the dead" in savasana is a great pose to do in bed. Yoga has been one of my personal favorite relaxation practices for many years. I find the practice calms my mind, lifts my spirit, helps release muscle tension and kinks, and aids in flexibility and strength.

Yoga is used in mainstream medicine for wellness regimens, in hospital disease management programs, and by psychologists for stressed-out and anxious clients. For sleep disorders, yoga is most beneficial for stress relief and combating fatigue. Author Indra Devi covers yoga's health perks: "You will be able to enjoy better sleep, a happier disposition, a clearer and calmer mind. You will learn how to build up your health and protect yourself against colds, fevers, constipation, headaches, fatigue, and other troubles. You will know what to do in order to remain youthful, vital and alert, regardless of your calendar-age; how to lose or gain weight; how to get rid of premature wrinkles, and keep a smooth skin and clear complexion."[107]

Undrugged **Tidbit: Yoga for Anxiety**

Get your *asana* on and toss antidepressant drugs! Just three yoga sessions per week boosts GABA levels, which improves mood and decreases anxiety.

CHAPTER 11

Drug-Induced Disease: Drugs, Herbs, and Supplements That Can Cause Insomnia

> The best and most efficient pharmacy is within your own system.
> —Robert C. Peale

Is my medication causing my insomnia? Insomnia can be a drug side effect, and any medication affecting the central nervous system can potentially sabotage your sleep. Assess your current medication list and nail down drugs with listed side effects of insomnia, sleep disruption or stimulation. For a more efficient and expedited process, have your favorite pharmacist conduct a medication review for you. I have helped countless patients over the years by performing a detailed medication reconciliation looking for issues like side effects, duplications, or other potential issues. Enlisting an expert eye is an excellent proactive health measure you should take advantage of. Your sleep solution may be as simple as adjusting medication timing, or could require physician intervention for dose adjustment or drug substitution to a non-stimulating medication, or removal of the drug altogether.

Prescription and Over-the-Counter Medications

The following is a condensed list of the *most common* stimulating drugs with the highest incidence of sleep disruption, increased nighttime awakenings, and disrupted REM sleep.[108]

Brain and central nervous system (CNS)

- ADHD medications: Dextroamphetamine, levoamphetamine, methamphetamine, methylphenidate
- Alzheimer's medications: donepezil, galantamine, rivastigmine
- Antidepressants: bupropion, citalopram, duloxetine, escitalopram, fluoxetine, fluvoxamine, isocarboxazid, moclobemide, paroxetine, phenelzine, reboxetine, sertraline, tranylcypromine, venlafaxine
- Appetite suppressants: naltrexone/bupropion (Contrave), phentermine, topiramate (Qsymia)
- Parkinson's medications: amantadine, biperiden, carbidopa, levodopa, rasagiline, selegiline

Heart and cardiovascular system

- ACE inhibitors: benazepril, captopril, enalapril, fosinopril, lisinopril, moexipril, perindopril, quinapril, ramipril, trandolapril
- Alpha-blockers: alfuzosin, doxazosin, prazosin, silodosin, terazosin, tamsulosin
- Antiarrhythmics: amiodarone, disopyramide, procainamide, quinidine
- Beta-blockers: atenolol, metoprolol, propranolol, and less with carvedilol, sotalol, timolol
- Diuretics or "water pills": chlorothiazide, chlorthalidone, hydrochlorothiazide
- Statins: atorvastatin, lovastatin, rosuvastatin, simvastatin

Lungs and inflammatory conditions

- Asthma medications: albuterol and theophylline
- Steroids: beclomethasone, budesonide, cortisone, flunisolide, fluticasone, methylprednisolone, mometasone, prednisone, prednisolone, triamcinolone

Other categories

- Hormones: DHEA and pregnenolone
- Nicotine patches/gum/inhalers/lozenges: Nicoderm, Nicorette, Nicotrol, Commit
- Thyroid medications: levothyroxine, thyroxine

Over-the-counter drugs

- Cough and cold drugs with decongestants: phenylephrine, pseudoephedrine
- Cough and cold drugs with alcohol: Coricidin HBP, Nyquil Cough, Theraflu Warming Relief
- Pain relief drugs with caffeine: Anacin, Caffedrine, Excedrin, Midol, Motrin Complete, NoDoz, Vivarin

Supplements and Herbs

During the day, you may benefit from boosted energy and mental clarity from many supplements and herbs. However, to avoid hindering your sleep, take the following supplements and herbs before lunch or take a decreased dose:[109]

Herbs

- Ashwaganda
- Chlorophyll
- Ginkgo Biloba
- Ginseng (*Panax ginseng* and *Panax quinquefolium*) and Siberian Ginseng (*Eleutherococcus senticosus*)
- Glucosamine/chondroitin
- Green tea

- Guarana
- Hoodia
- Kola Nut
- Reishi mushroom
- Rhodiola
- Stinging nettle
- St. John's Wort
- Tongkat ali
- Herbs with diuretic effects: celery seed, cleavers, dandelion, elderflowers, horsetail, juniper, nettle leaf, parsley, yarrow

Supplements

- Carnitine and Acetyl-L-carnitine
- High-potency multivitamins
- Phenylalanine
- Sam-e (S-adenosylmethionine)
- Taurine
- Tyrosine
- High doses of the following: alpha lipoic acid; B vitamins, especially B6 and B12; CoQ10; fish oil and krill oil

Is your sleep interrupted by nightmares that leave you stressed out and exhausted? Nightmares create intense feelings of inescapable fear, terror, distress, and extreme anxiety, and may make you feel like you are suffocating, falling off a building to a certain death, or even struggling to scream or wake up. Were you aware there is a documented connection between nightmares and drugs? I found this intriguing, as this side effect is not typically highlighted in pharmacy school curriculum or even in physician interactions with pharmaceutical sales forces. Many medications, hormones, herbs, and supplements are known to alter dreams, making them more vivid. Women and children are more prone to these effects. Drugs that can cause nightmares include:[110]

- Alzheimer's drugs: donepezil, memantine, rivastigmine, tacrine
- Anesthesia drugs: isoflurane, midazolam, thiopental
- Antibiotic drugs: ciprofloxacin, erythromycin

Dr. Lori Arnold, PharmD

- Blood pressure drugs: atenolol, betaxolol, bisoprolol, guanethidine, labetalol, propranolol, reserpine
- Cholesterol drugs: atorvastatin, fluvastatin, pravastatin, simvastatin
- Depression drugs: citalopram, clomipramine, fluoxetine, mirtazapine
- Epilepsy drugs: gabapentin, tiagabine, valproic acid
- Hormones: DHEA, testosterone
- Parkinson's drugs: amantadine, bromocriptine, levodopa, pergolide, rasagiline, selegiline
- Sleep drugs: zolpidem
- Smoking cessation drugs: varenicline

CHAPTER 12

Replenish and Restore: Drug Alternatives

> The reason one vitamin can cure so many illnesses is because a deficiency of one vitamin can cause many illnesses.
> —Dr. Andrew Saul

I have equipped you with an arsenal of useful tools and tricks for your sleep hygiene *readjust*. I hope you were able to identify possible sleep-zapping factors, bringing you closer to pinpointing the root cause of your insomnia. Several *undrugged* lifestyle suggestions are great substitutes for chemical sleep aids and can help set your trajectory to restoring healthy sleep habits. Sometimes, however, simple habit modification will not remedy insomnia if the underlying issue is a hormonal imbalance or neurotransmitter deficiency created by other drugs. *Replenish and restore* provides additional valuable drug alternatives when a more targeted hormonal or biochemical approach is warranted.

Undrugged Sleepy-Time Supplements, Herbs, and Aromatherapy

Long before pharmaceutical companies started selling chemical sleep aids, holistic remedies were a mainstay. Make Hippocrates proud by returning to "old-school" healing treatments. Your first-line insomnia defense should be a multimodal combination of healthier sleep hygiene habits and safer drug-free natural alternatives. Your goal is to *eliminate the cause* of insomnia, not merely dab on a little superglue and hope it holds. Don't forget, sleeping pills mask symptoms. Insomnia may actually be a symptom produced by your body's internal alert system, signaling an underlying vitamin, mineral, or hormonal deficiency. Common nutrient deficiencies often seen with disturbed sleep include niacin, magnesium, copper, iron, tryptophan, and vitamin B6.[111]

Intelligent insomnia treatment employs a *nutraceutical* approach, targeting potential nutrient deficiencies. Nutraceuticals are high-quality, pharmaceutical-grade nutritional supplements, manufactured by reputable companies who adhere to quality and safe manufacturing practices. Many of these companies submit voluntary data to the FDA for purity testing. Supplement dosing is highly individualized. Therefore, always start low and go slow. If a small dose works, don't assume doubling the dose will give you twice the effect. Like pharmaceutical drugs, higher doses of nutraceuticals can also be riddled with increased side effects. In my professional opinion, a one-size-fits-all approach is not safe or effective and can leave you more tired and frustrated after countless unsuccessful attempts. Rather than donning a "Google MD" degree, find a skilled practitioner who can customize a sleep treatment protocol specifically designed for you and your needs. By doing this, you are building a safety net to catch any interactions or issues, especially if mixing with antidepressants, blood pressure drugs, other sleep aids, or alcohol. This section furnishes you with the *undrugged* collection of suggested supplements, herbals, and aromatherapy remedies to help you fall asleep and stay asleep with fewer side effects than drugs.[112] Each nutraceutical is broken into an easy-to-access format for quick reference, to include description and mechanism of action; sources of depletion; safe use, including cautions and side effects; and dosing recommendations.

Nutraceuticals

Melatonin

Melatonin is a hormone and antioxidant made in the brain and digestive tract that helps regulate the body's internal clock. Some forms of insomnia are linked to melatonin depletion. In chapter 2, recall pharma tapped into the nutraceutical arena by attempting to sell an overpriced version of melatonin. Don't be fooled, and don't waste your money. To boost levels, an over-the-counter, synthetic melatonin supplement may be used, offering the exact chemical structure as natural melatonin. When replacing melatonin, it is imperative to add adequate vitamin B6, as B6 efficiently drives hormonal production. If your sleeplessness is caused by low levels of melatonin, studies show melatonin will help lessen time taken to fall asleep, provide higher quality sleep, and increase total sleep time.[113] Melatonin is a favorite among jet-lagged travelers who frequently need help adjusting to new time zones.

Sources of depletion: Melatonin production decreases as you age, which explains why you have more trouble sleeping the older you get. Certain drugs block melatonin production, including acetaminophen, ibuprofen, naproxen, and aspirin. Be especially cautious with aspirin, as 75 percent of melatonin production can be hindered with just one dose of aspirin. If continuing any of these medications, take your last dose prior to dinner.

Safe use: Short-term use limited to a few weeks is safe; however, evidence on long-term use is lacking. Experts warn using melatonin long-term may cause your body to adjust by decreasing natural melatonin production. Basically, it becomes a "use it or lose it" situation, where the more synthetic melatonin you take, the less your body has to produce. If you teach your body to create less endogenous melatonin, you will be forced to continue taking synthetic melatonin to make up for the depletion—you do not want to create this situation.

Prolonged use or very high doses may cause toxicity, headaches, nightmares, increased depression, sex hormone suppression, and even infertility. Due to melatonin's immune system stimulation, avoid use if you have an autoimmune disease or immune-related cancers like lymphoma and leukemia. Avoid while pregnant, lactating, or attempting to conceive. Avoid if taking other sleep aids, seizure drugs, SSRI or MAOI antidepressants, or corticosteroids. The most common side effects include nausea, headache, and dizziness. Some people have reported vivid dreams or discontinued treatment due to nightmares. With all sleep aids, even supplements and herbs, allow at least eight hours for sleep to lessen morning grogginess.

Dosing: Dose range is 0.3 mg to 6 mg, taken in a dark room thirty to sixty minutes prior to bedtime. Start low dose and titrate to optimal effect. Females should always initiate at 0.3 mg, the lowest effective dose. For immediate sleep-inducing results, take a 3 mg rapid-acting sublingual tab, thirty minutes prior to bedtime. For help staying asleep, take a 0.3 mg (300 mcg) extended-release tab, at least four full hours prior to bedtime. Timing is crucial with extended-release, as maximum effectiveness is only achieved prior to your body making natural melatonin at night. For best results, take with 10 mg vitamin B6, 1,000 mcg vitamin B12 (methylcobalamin), 225 mg magnesium, and 11 mg zinc.

Avoid nightly doses and try limiting use to one to two times weekly. If taking melatonin at very high doses (greater than 6 mg) or for more than two weeks with little or no effect, reassess your treatment plan, as it is highly unlikely melatonin depletion is the root cause of your sleeplessness. Do not continue to increase to higher doses, as this will increase the likelihood for side effects.

Magnesium

Magnesium is crucial for optimal health and is required for over three hundred enzymatic reactions in your body, making it one of my personal *undrugged* favorite picks. Approximately 75 percent of Americans have some level of magnesium deficiency. Magnesium deficiency can manifest as anxiety, depression, muscle weakness, fatigue, eye twitching, anorexia, poor memory, confusion, anger, nervousness, rapid pulse, and insomnia. You may not even realize a multitude of your symptoms and system-wide dysfunction may be directly related to low levels of this vital nutrient.[114] Magnesium supplementation is essential to sleep, as it acts as a natural tranquilizer that helps induce sleep and relaxes nerve impulses.[115]

Sources of depletion: Many drugs decrease magnesium levels, including diuretics, digoxin, cholesterol drugs, steroids, hormone therapy, insulin, antibiotics, acid blockers, and alcohol.

Safe use: Often referred to as "nature's calcium channel blocker," magnesium naturally lowers blood pressure by helping your heart function more efficiently. If taking blood pressure drugs, monitor your blood pressure and heart rate closely and speak to your doctor about a possible drug dose reduction. Be sure to seek medical approval prior to taking additional magnesium if you have liver or kidney disease. Higher doses may cause diarrhea; therefore, reduce dose to bowel tolerance. You can do this by identifying the dose that causes loose stools and reducing this dose by one tablet or 100 to 200 mg.

Dosing: Start dose low at 200 to 600 mg nightly, taken one to two hours prior to bedtime. My *undrugged* favorite is magnesium glycinate, as it is well tolerated, with the additional benefit of nighttime relaxation. Magnesium gluconate and lactate forms are also well tolerated. Magnesium oxide, sulfate, and hydroxide cause more diarrhea, especially if the dose exceeds 600 mg. For maximum effectiveness, take with 50 mg vitamin B6. To further calm and enhance relaxation, combine magnesium with calcium in a one-to-two ratio, starting with 250 mg magnesium and 500 mg calcium.

5-HTP (5-hydroxytryptophan)

5-HTP is crucial for the chemical reaction that creates serotonin and melatonin.[116] When used for sleep, 5-HTP helps reduce the time it takes to fall asleep and increases the duration and quality of sleep.[117] Use of 5-HTP can also soothe the nervous system, enhance feelings of well-being, help control appetite, enhance libido, and regulate blood pressure. 5-HTP has also shown to improve restful sleep in children who frequently wake from sleep terrors. Symptoms of 5-HTP deficiency are the same as those seen with serotonin depletion—negative disposition, depression, irritability, anger, feeling anxious or fearful, or having obsessive thoughts and compulsions.

Safe use: Avoid use if taking corticosteroids. Avoid SSRI or MAOI antidepressants, as the combined use increases risk for "serotonin syndrome," characterized by nausea, sweating, headache, and increased blood pressure. Notify your doctor if any of these symptoms occur. High 5-HTP doses increase side effect risk, and doses exceeding 200 mg can raise the stress hormone, cortisol, further sabotaging sleep efforts.

Dr. Lori Arnold, PharmD

Dosing: Dose range is 50 to 200 mg, taken at least one hour before bedtime. Start with lowest dose and titrate to optimal effect. When beginning 5-HTP supplementation, mild nausea is common and typically subsides after a few days of use. For maximum effectiveness, take with 50 mg vitamin B6 and 1,000 mcg vitamin B12 (methylcobalamin).

GABA (gamma-aminobutyric acid)

GABA is an amino acid and a neurotransmitter that blocks nerve overfiring, thus aiding with the generation of healthy sleep brain waves.[118] Depletion of GABA manifests physically as insomnia, anxiety, stress, agitation, panic attacks, emotional outbursts, intense food cravings for carbohydrate-rich foods like sugar or starchy treats, and cravings for alcohol or drugs to calm and relax. GABA is extremely beneficial for stress-induced insomnia, as it induces relaxation and sleep, helps increase growth hormone, reduces hypoglycemia (which can wake you in the middle of the night), lowers blood pressure, relaxes muscles, and restores calmness to the brain.[119]

Safe use: Seek medical approval prior to taking GABA if you have liver or kidney disease. Avoid if you are pregnant or lactating. Avoid in children younger than six years old. Do not combine with anxiety drugs or alcohol.

Dosing: Dose range is 250 to 500 mg, taken thirty to sixty minutes before bedtime. Start with lowest dose and titrate to optimal effect. For quicker onset, take sublingual GABA. Since GABA is very effective at promoting drowsiness, it is best taken while in bed. For maximum effectiveness, take with 50 mg vitamin B6.

Vitamin B6 (pyridoxine)

Vitamin B6 is a cofactor in over a hundred essential enzymatic reactions, including those that increase sleep hormones and neurotransmitters. This often overlooked powerhouse drives biochemical pathways that produce melatonin, serotonin, GABA, and dopamine and helps boost magnesium levels. Depletion of vitamin B6 often manifests as brain-related symptoms, including sleep disturbances, lethargy, decreased alertness, and depression. Gauge yourself for B6 depletion by using a simple "dream test." Based on dream recollection, add B6 if you are unable to dream; if you have trouble remembering dreams; or if your dreams are stressful, weird, or frightening. Studies show that supplementation with vitamin B6 improves dream recall and overall quality of dreams.[120]

Sources of depletion: Your body's ability to utilize vitamin B6 decreases as you age, thus necessitating supplementation. Drugs that deplete critical stores of vitamin B6 include oral contraceptives, antidepressants, decongestants, diuretics, cortisone, L-dopa, and theophylline. In addition, vitamin B6 is depleted with exposure to alcohol, smoking, food additives (tartrazine, yellow #5), chemicals, pesticides, and excessive protein intake.

Safe use: Doses greater than 500 mg daily increase side effects. Symptoms of toxicity include tingling in the hands and feet, loss of muscle coordination, and gait disturbances. Because vitamin B6 is water soluble, most symptoms can be reversed once B6 dose is lowered or discontinued. A nerve toxicity called peripheral neuropathy may occur at high doses in excess of 2,000 mg daily. Avoid if you take levodopa for Parkinson's disease. In order to avoid creating other B vitamin deficiencies, it is advisable to take vitamin B6 as part of a B complex vitamin.

Dosing: Dose range is 50 to 200 mg twice daily with meals. Make sure to take the last dose with dinner, as B vitamins can be stimulating for some. Your liver can only process 50 mg at a time. Therefore, spread doses greater than 50 mg throughout the day. Utilize the "dream test" to help target your dose requirement.[121] You will know you have reached your nutrient "sweet spot" when your dreams become more frequent and pleasant.

If you approach the maximum 500 mg daily without improvement in dream recollection, switch to the active and more absorbable form called pyridoxal 5-phosphate (P5P). Dose range of P5P is 25 to 100 mg daily with meals, which is equivalent to about 100 to 125 mg of regular vitamin B6. Stress depletes B vitamins. Therefore, be aware you may need to increase your dose during stressful times.

Dr. Lori Arnold, PharmD

Valerian Root (*Valeriana officinalis*)

The herb valerian is a folk remedy that has been used for hundreds of years to calm and sedate by helping the brain release GABA. For insomnia, valerian may increase deep sleep, lessen time taken to fall asleep, decrease nighttime awakenings, and improve total sleep quality.[122] It has also been effectively used for anxiety and depression due to its ability to calm fear, reduce restlessness, and lessen aggression.[123]

Safe use: Limit valerian use to less than thirty consecutive days. Approximately 10 percent of people experience increased energy with valerian, which could hinder sleep efforts. Do not combine with antihistamines, antidepressants, antianxiety agents, other sleeping drugs, or alcohol. Avoid if you are pregnant or breastfeeding. Common side effects include headache, itchiness, dizziness, and gastrointestinal upset.

Dosing: Dose ranges from 600 to 900 mg, taken sixty minutes before bedtime. Valerian is available as capsules, tablets, liquids, tinctures, extracts, and teas. If using a valerian tincture, take fresh root tincture that is 0.8 percent valerenic acid. The capsule or tablet form is preferred, as many find the flavor of the tincture and tea bitter and unappealing.

Undrugged Drug Substitutions

Hopefully, you've been able to identify specific sleep sabotages throughout this book. Some of these conditions have targeted solutions. Here is a brief compilation of suggestions for specific sleep-related issues.

Caffeine-induced insomnia: Combine 100 mg *valerian root* with 30 to 120 mg of *hops extract* before bedtime. Although hops can be found in beer, pounding a beer before bed won't give you the same effect. Known for its calming effects, hops extract is a mild sedative often used for anxiety and insomnia.[124]

Restless legs syndrome (RLS): Pharma will not like my *undrugged* RLS solution after it has poured billions of dollars into the promotion of chemical RLS products. If you suffer from RLS or nighttime leg cramps, take 50 mg vitamin B6, 400 mcg folic acid, and 225 mg magnesium at least an hour before bedtime.[125] Have your doctor check your iron levels. If you have low to normal ferritin levels, consider adding iron supplementation per your practitioner's guidance.[126] Studies show many people have eliminated RLS using this combination.

Anxiety-induced insomnia: Ditch benzodiazepine sleep agents. My *undrugged* preferred anxiety drug substitution is the product GABA Calm, made by Source Naturals. GABA Calm contains GABA, magnesium, glycine, N-acetyl L-tyrosine, and taurine. For insomnia, take one tab after dinner and repeat another one to two tabs thirty to sixty minutes before bedtime. To help calm emotions during anxiety-related stressful daytime issues, take one to two tabs between meals as needed. Another of my favorite products is PharmaGABA, made by Designs for Health. PharmaGABA contains 200 mg of GABA. For maximum benefit, chew two tablets thirty to sixty minutes prior to bedtime.

"Tired-and-Wired" Insomnia: This is my *undrugged* "preferred choice" zolpidem replacement for those suffering from "tired-and-wired insomnia" and bedtime monkey mind. Insomnitol Chewables, made by Designs for Health, has worked very effectively for many of my clients. This product calms brain activity to help you fall asleep and stay asleep throughout the night. Insomnitol contains all the good stuff, including vitamin B6, inositol, L-theanine, 5-HTP, and melatonin. For maximum benefit, chew two tablets thirty to sixty minutes prior to bedtime. My personal zolpidem-replacement sleep cocktail includes two tablets of Insomnitol Chewables with two tablets of PharmaGABA, taken at least sixty minutes prior to bedtime. I like to swap GABA Calm and PharmaGABA every so often if I feel my regular regimen isn't working as well as I'd like it to. Make sure you only take one of the GABA products, not both. I also take 400 to 600 mg of magnesium glycinate every night. To obtain Designs for Health products, go to www.healyourselfbeautiful.com, and click on the tab for "products."

Dr. Lori Arnold, PharmD

Herbal Teas

Sipping an evening cup of non-caffeinated, herbal tea before bedtime is soothing and promotes sleepiness by raising your body temperature. One cup is good; two isn't necessarily better. Liquid consumption should be limited for the last one to two hours before bed to avoid urgent bladder pressure that can disrupt your sleep. The following are a few sleepy-time relaxing herbal teas you may incorporate into your nightly regimen:

Chamomile (*Matricaria chamomilla* **and** *recutita***)**: Chamomile helps you chill out. It eases insomnia and enhances sedation and even calms restlessness and irritability in children. A constituent of chamomile, *apigenin*, binds to GABA in the brain, creating a mild antianxiety effect similar to the prescription drug alprazolam (Xanax).[127] It also has been found to increase glycine, a chemical that relaxes the nervous system and acts like a mild sedative.[128]

Passionflower (*Passiflora incarnata***)**: Herbalists utilize passionflower to help ease mental worry, overwork, and nervous exhaustion. For sleep, passionflower effectively induces drowsiness by calming and relaxing the nervous system. As a bonus, passionflower's antispasmodic properties also help relax blood vessels, digestion, and breathing.[129]

Decaffeinated green tea: Decaf green tea contains the amino acid L-theanine, which has been shown to reduce stress and promote sedation. It does so by calming the nervous system, thus reducing alertness and slowing down brain wave activity. L-theanine's actions improves total sleep quality, helping you feel more rested upon awakening.[130]

Undrugged Tidbit: Sleep Easy with Herbal Tea

Replace low-dose prescription antianxiety drugs with chamomile tea. Apigenin, a constituent of chamomile tea, binds to brain GABA creating a mild antianxiety response.

Aromatherapy: Applying Essential Oils

When I create an integrative medication summary for my clients, I always incorporate some component of aromatherapy into their regimens and treatment plans. Aromatherapy is the clinical application of plant-derived essential oils for health benefits. To ensure optimal response, only use high-quality essential oils that are guaranteed pesticide-free, excipient-free, and unadulterated. To further instill confidence in a product's efficacy, choose essential oil brands that have been tested in clinical trials by major teaching institutions or hospitals. I discourage jumping blindly into the Pinterest-driven, social media aromatherapy-hype by attempting home study if utilizing oils as an adjunct to medical treatment or if you are trying to remove the drug completely. Most traditionally trained physicians will quickly pooh-pooh your oil plan if you can't back it up with medical literature or impressive case studies; anecdotal hearsay doesn't hold much weight when trying to convince most medical professionals. Instead, assume the role of a savvy, informed consumer on this one. Just because oils are considered "natural" does not automatically mean they are "safe." To assure your safety, I find it most effective to work with a holistic practitioner or coach who is credentialed in aromatherapy. As is the case with any natural treatment or drug, just because a couple drops of oil work well, doesn't automatically mean ten to fifteen drops will work better. Higher doses greatly increase the likelihood of new and bothersome side effects, and in some cases, exceeding the recommended dose may create an entirely opposite effect than originally intended.

This section provides suggestions for safe and appropriate, sleep-promoting essential oils. All of my recommendations utilize topical or inhaled administration routes. For topical administration, many oils can be applied directly to the skin, which is called "neat" application. Oils may also be diluted with a "carrier oil," like coconut oil, almond oil, jojoba oil, or other soothing oil bases. Some oils require dilution prior to application due to higher irritant properties. Combining diluted essentials oils with techniques like massage or therapeutic touch is an outstanding way to promote restful sleep and enhance a calming and relaxing experience. When using inhalation for application, you may sniff or waft aroma directly from the vial or diffuse into the room. Investing in an oil diffuser is highly encouraged, as the nebulization of essential oils disperses a fine mist covering hundreds of square feet in seconds. Using oils in this simple manner keeps oils suspended in room air, allowing you to reap the healing benefits of the aromatherapy for several hours.

Adding essential oils to your evening regimen enhances the likelihood of achieving more restful and restorative sleep. The following essential oils have shown benefit for sleep and relaxation:

Lavender Oil (*Lavandula angustifolia*)

For centuries, lavender has been used to help promote relaxation and sedation and to lower stress and anxiety, and it's now being used by many hospitals to help aid with sleep.[131] One study showed insomniacs had a 50 percent improvement in symptoms after sleeping in a room with lavender aroma. Exercise caution, as too much lavender can induce stimulation, thus sabotaging sleep efforts.[132]

Suggested use: Use one or more of these techniques:

- *Topical.* Apply one to two drops of oil to temples, reflex points, or on wrists. Place one to two drops in palms of hands and inhale aroma deeply, using deep breathing techniques. Massage one to two drops to the back or bottom of feet at bedtime or dilute three to five drops with a carrier oil and massage over entire body.
- *Inhaled.* Using an oil diffuser, diffuse three to four drops of oil at bedtime or inhale aroma directly from vial. Diffuse in bedroom for a minimum of two hours before lying down to sleep. Combine with calming music, solfeggio, nature sounds, prayer, or meditation.
- *Other applications.* Sprinkle one to two drops of oil on your pillowcase. Create a *relaxation bath* by adding one half to one cup Epsom salts and three to five drops of lavender oil to warm water. Epsom salt is an excellent magnesium source that absorbs directly into your body to help calm and relax muscles, and the warm bath water helps adjust your body to the appropriate temperature that encourages sleepiness.

***Undrugged* Tidbit: Effective Essential Oils to Aid with Sleep**
Essential oils are essential for sleep! Compared to conventional nursing interventions, cardiac intensive care patients had decreased anxiety and improved sleep quality when exposed to an aromatherapy blend of lavender, Roman chamomile, and neroli (*Citrus aurantium*).[133]

Juniper Berry Oil (*Juniperus communis*)

Juniper berry oil is both renewing and equalizing and is used for spiritual and physical purification. Emotionally, juniper berry helps you quell feelings of fear and anxiety, which contribute to nightmares and disturbing dreams that may increase frequent awakenings and disruption of sleep patterns.[134]

Suggested use: Use one or more of these techniques:

- *Topical.* Apply one two drops of oil to forehead or behind ears before bed. You may dilute with coconut oil, if desired.
- *Inhaled.* Using an oil diffuser, diffuse three to four drops of oil at bedtime or inhale directly from vial. I like to mix my own calming potion in my diffuser by blending juniper berry with lavender, bergamot, and geranium.

Sweet Marjoram Oil (*Origanum majorana*)

Sweet marjoram oil promotes peace and sleep. For sedation, it calms and induces relaxation and helps relieve anxiety and nervous stress. For mood, it uplifts and generates happiness during times of anger or sadness. When applied topically for body relaxation, it helps soothe and ease muscle tension, spasms, and stiff joints.[135]

Suggested use: Use one or more of these techniques:

- *Topical.* Apply one two three drops of oil over your heart before bed. You may dilute three to five drops with a carrier oil, like coconut oil, and massage over sore muscles.
- *Inhaled.* Using an oil diffuser, diffuse three to four drops of oil at bedtime or inhale directly from the vial.

Roman Chamomile Oil (*Chamaemelum nobile* or *Anthemis nobilis*)

In ancient Rome, soldiers used Roman chamomile before battle for empowerment, to clear mental blocks, and to improve courage. For insomnia and meditation, it is calming and relaxing and effective at eliminating highly charged emotions, like irritability, anxiety, and nervousness. When applied topically for body relaxation, it helps relieve muscle tension and restless legs.[136]

Suggested use: Use one or more of these techniques:

- *Topical.* Apply three to six drops of oil over stomach or one drop over forehead or behind ears before bed. You may dilute three to five drops with a carrier oil and apply directly to tight or sore areas.
- *Inhaled.* Using an oil diffuser, diffuse three to four drops of oil at bedtime or inhale directly from the vial.
- *Other application.* Add three to six drops of oil to warm bathwater before bed.

Patchouli Oil (*Pogostemon cablin*)

Patchouli oil is considered grounding and stabilizing and is energetically connected to security, stability, and spirituality. Patchouli can be used alone or mixed with other oils to enhance prayer and meditation. It beautifully compliments mind-body-spirit practices like yoga and tai chi and energy work like Reiki. It helps calm fears and eases tension and helps release you from obsessive monkey-mind, chattering thoughts that prevent you from falling asleep. Exercise caution with patchouli, as it is a sedative at low doses and a stimulant at high doses.[137]

Suggested use: Use one or more of these techniques:

- *Topical.* Apply one to three drops of oil to bottom of feet or below the navel before bed. You may dilute with a carrier oil, like coconut oil, if desired.
- *Inhaled.* Using a diffuser, diffuse three to four drops of oil at bedtime or inhale directly from vial.

Sandalwood Oil (*Santalum album*)

Since ancient times, sandalwood oil has been used for grounding and in spiritual applications to help restore peace to the heart. For insomnia, it helps quiet internal mind chatter that keeps you awake during the night. For emotions, it can be used for stress, depression, and low self-esteem and may help improve overall emotional balance.[138]

Suggested use: Use one or more of these techniques:

- *Topical.* Apply one to two drops of oil to forehead or behind ears before bed. You may dilute with a carrier oil, like coconut oil, if desired.
- *Inhaled.* Using a diffuser, diffuse three to four drops of oil at bedtime or inhale directly from vial.

Undrugged **Tidbit: Stimulating Essential Oils**

Do *not* use these essential oils at bedtime, as they may cause stimulation and wakefulness—rosemary (*Rosmarinus officinalis*), lemon (*Citrus limon*), jasmine (*Jasminum officinale*), and peppermint (*Mentha piperita*).[139] I *do*, however, encourage you to utilize these oils in the morning to help refresh and renew your energy levels for waking hours.

Dr. Lori Arnold, PharmD

Along with the *undrugged* good sleep hygiene habits I have provided, essential oils are an excellent adjunct to any routine. I handpicked just a few essential oils that help enhance relaxation and calmness, but many more oils are beneficial for these purposes. Several reputable essential oil companies have even created customized sleep blends incorporating effective sedative and calming oils. As with all natural treatments, you will need to experiment in order to identify what works best for you and your needs. Every individual experiences varied reactions and emotions to each aroma or specific oil application. For instance, I may emotionally connect with the aroma of jasmine oil, but you, on the other hand, may find the smell of jasmine offensive to your senses.

You should have a little fun combining oils by creating your own personalized diffuser blends. When combined, you will create a wonderful "aromatherapy cocktail." I have simplified this by creating a few *undrugged* diffuser "sleep tonics" and insomnia potions:

Undrugged Sleep Tonics for Your Aromatherapy Diffuser:

Sleep blend to "count blessings not sheep for sleep": Diffuse together four drops lavender oil, two drops bergamot oil, two drops juniper berry oil, and two drops ylang ylang oil.

Sleep blend to ease stress: Diffuse together three drops vetiver oil, three drops lavender oil, three drops sandalwood oil, and two drops ylang ylang oil.

Sleep blend to ease headaches: Diffuse together three drops Roman chamomile oil, three drops lavender oil, and three drops sweet marjoram oil.

Sleep blend to ease snoring: Diffuse together three drops thyme oil, three drops cedarwood oil and three drops sweet marjoram oil.

Undrugged **Tidbit: Do You Snore Like a Freight Train?**

Several prescription drugs make snoring worse. To help ease snoring and strained breathing, mix one drop cypress oil with two drops coconut oil or any carrier oil and apply topically over your throat before bed. Then mix one drop thyme oil with four drops coconut oil and apply topically to your big toe. Transform your snore train to *The Little Engine That Could*, quietly chugging your way to snooze *Little Engine That Could* land in no time!

CHAPTER 13

Refresh: Healing with Food

Let your food be your medicine and let your medicine be your food.
—Hippocrates

Food is a potent sleep influencer. Insomnia lurks beneath complex meals with multiple ingredients, very spicy or rich foods, refined sugar, alcohol, coffee and tea, large portions, late-night dinners, and heavy bedtime snacks. Feasting on lumberjack-sized portions and improper meal timing will inflict a deluge of digestive woes, miserably lingering for several hours—sometimes even the entire night. *Refresh* gives you wiser food choices by helping identify sleep-boosting and sleep-sabotaging foods. Incorporating this information as a general nighttime food and snacking guide will improve your ability to fall asleep and stay asleep.

Sleep-Boosting Foods

It is time to "rest and digest." Your good sleep insurance policy begins by forgoing rich and heavy dinners and by consuming all meals at least two to three hours prior to bedtime. The contents of your dinner plate should be light, restricting animal meat or fish to three to four ounces, organic vegetables should be consumed in abundance, and a small serving of complex carbohydrates should be added to appropriately round off a nutritious meal. Instead of going to bed starving, grab a healthy snack that supports relaxation and sleep. Some nutrition experts claim that organic foods produce sweeter dreams, while high fat or carbohydrate-heavy junk foods result in nightmares. Restful sleep can be significantly affected by the content of your dreams.

Select nighttime foods containing nutrients that boost sleep hormones and neurotransmitters. Optimal choices are highest in natural melatonin, serotonin, tryptophan, calcium, magnesium, potassium, and vitamin B6 and B12. Bedtime is not a time to be "carbophobic," especially if you are struggling to sleep. Add complex carbohydrates to your plate and reap the health and sleep benefits. You can opt to go "all natural" by only utilizing food as your sleep aid, or you can achieve maximum benefit by combining vitamin or herbal supplementation with smart snacking choices. Either way, through trial and error, you will find what works best for you and be *pleasantly* snoozing in no time.[140]

Sleep-Boosting Foods

These foods are highest in sleep-promoting nutrients, with several foods containing multiple beneficial vitamins and minerals. The rule of thumb with all snacks: Consume at least an hour before bedtime.

- Brewer's yeast
- Dairy products (milk, yogurt, cottage cheese, cheese)
- Dates
- Eggs
- Fruit (apples, avocado, banana, blueberries, pineapple, raspberries)
- Goji berries
- Honey
- Hummus (chickpeas)
- Nuts and seeds (almonds, cashews, chia seeds, flaxseeds, peanuts, pistachios, pumpkin and sunflower seeds, walnuts)
- Oats
- Organic popcorn
- Poultry (chicken and turkey)
- Seafood (cod, crab, halibut, lobster, salmon, sardines, shrimp, tuna)

- Tart cherry juice
- Vegetables (butternut squash, orange bell peppers, spinach, sweet potato)

Sleep-Boosting Spices and Herbs

Frequently add these spices and herbs to foods as they boost production of sleep hormones and neurotransmitters.

- Basil
- Coriander
- Dill
- Fenugreek
- Mustard seeds
- Nutmeg
- Oregano
- Parsley
- Saffron
- Sage
- Spirulina

Undrugged Favorite **Food Choices**:

I encourage you to add the following foods to your evening regimen to assure you are choosing fail-safe, choice, sleep-enhancing foods.

Tart Cherry Juice: Tart cherry juice is one of the richest food sources of melatonin. It contains phytomelatonin, a plant nutrient that helps regulate sleep-wake cycles. A 2012 study showed volunteers consuming tart cherry juice for seven days had significantly elevated melatonin and improved sleep quality and duration.[141] As a bonus, it has shown benefit in balancing mood, managing stress, improving immune system function, and helping promote sleep in children who wake frequently. One cup of tart cherry juice or one-eighths cup dried tart cherries is roughly equivalent to 0.3 mg of melatonin supplement.[142]

How to use. Drink two eight-ounce servings daily, one serving between 8:00 to 10:00 a.m. and the second serving one to two hours before bedtime. Since this juice is *tart*, you can improve taste by diluting in water with a touch of stevia and a drop of vanilla.

Oats: Oats should not be reserved only for breakfast, as oats are rich in melatonin, magnesium, and potassium. A warm bowl of oatmeal before bed is a delicious comfort food. The higher carbohydrate content of oats helps elevate blood sugar, thus shuttling tryptophan into your brain. If you struggle with weight issues or blood sugar conditions like diabetes, you should opt for other food options due to the potential to increase blood sugar.
How to use. Select a high-quality, gluten-free, steel-cut variety. Limit your portion to a quarter cup dry oats. Add warm milk or almond milk to help boost the relaxation effect.

Almonds: Almonds are high in magnesium, calcium, and melatonin, which promote sleep and muscle relaxation. The protein in almonds helps stabilize blood sugar, and the healthy unsaturated fat content boosts heart health and aids in brain functioning.
How to use. Portion control is the key. Going nuts on nuts can create considerable indigestion, and the high fat content of excessive quantities can be difficult to digest. Always choose raw and unsalted varieties, as roasted and flavored varieties contain unhealthy fats, high sodium and undesirable chemicals. A portion size is equivalent to twenty-three almonds, about one ounce, or one tablespoon of almond butter.

Bananas: Bananas are often thought of as a source of energy or as a postexercise recovery food, but they are also excellent for sleep-enhancement. Bananas contain the "magic sleep trio" of magnesium, potassium, and tryptophan. Banana's high magnesium and potassium concentration aids in muscle relaxation and helps prevent muscle cramping, and vitamin B6 helps convert tryptophan into melatonin, which helps you fall asleep faster.
How to use. Don't go ape crazy with a jumbo-sized banana. Opt for a medium banana on the "greener" unripe side. The ripe bananas with brown spots can have up to double the sugar content of an unripe banana. Simply peel and eat!

Dr. Lori Arnold, PharmD

Complex carbs: Complex carbohydrates maximize L-tryptophan in the brain, aiding in the production of serotonin and melatonin.[143] People who consume quality whole food carbohydrates, not refined junk processed products, are invariably calm, rarely depressed, and able to sleep more soundly. One study showed insomniacs who ate foods high in tryptophan with complex carbohydrates had improvements in all sleep measurements, equivalent to taking a tryptophan supplement.[144]

Select complex carbohydrates from healthier sources, avoiding exposure to overly processed, refined grain products. The following foods should be incorporated into your dinner. Vegetables and beans, including asparagus, black-eyed peas, black beans, broccoli, Brussels sprouts, cabbage, cauliflower, chickpeas, green peas, kidney beans, lentils, potatoes, pumpkin, squash, sweet potatoes, yams, and zucchini. Preferred grain choices include barley, brown rice, wild rice, kamut, oatmeal, and quinoa. If you are intolerant or allergic to gluten, avoid whole wheat products. Apples and berries are acceptable fruit choices, as they contain the least amount of fruit sugar and the lowest glycemic index.

How to use. Consume with dinner or as a snack at least an hour prior to bedtime. Exercise strict portion control, as larger quantities can contribute to weight gain. A typical vegetable portion would be one cup raw vegetables or one-half cup cooked vegetables. A fruit portion is one medium apple or one-half cup chopped berries. A grain or bean portion is one-half cup.

Undrugged **Tidbit: Sleep-Promoting Nighttime Snacks:**

- Small organic apple with small handful of pumpkin seeds
- 1/2 cup raspberries with 6 ounces plain nonfat Greek yogurt
- Brown rice crackers with almond butter
- 1/4 cup plain oatmeal with one small mashed banana
- One organic brown rice cake with a tomato slice and slice of turkey breast
- One scoop whey protein powder with 1/2 banana and almond milk
- Hummus or eggplant hummus and veggies like cucumber, broccoli, and carrots

- Banana nut "soft serve dessert": Pulse blend a frozen banana for several minutes and add a small handful of chopped peanuts or 1 tablespoon nut butter. Mix well. May serve with cinnamon for added flavor.

Undrugged Tidbit: Restore Calm with Schisandra Berries

Schisandra berries (*Schisandra chinensis*) are powerful berries used by Chinese herbalists to calm the spirit and aid with insomnia, memory recall, and concentration. The astringent property is useful for treating frequent urination, nocturnal emissions, diarrhea, and excessive sweating.[145] Dried Schisandra berries can be found in Chinese groceries and medicine shops. You can safely consume up to 3 grams of dried berries daily. Schisandra supplements, standardized to schizandrins, is dosed at 1 to 3 grams daily.[87]

Sleep-Sabotaging Foods

To be snoozing in no time, you know what and when to eat. However, you also have to practice avoidance of the dreaded sleep-sabotaging foods. Continuing nighttime indulgences of foods listed in this section may keep you hitched to zolpidem for life—and this is one marriage you don't want to continue for the long haul. Discipline yourself to adjust your habits, and trust that the health benefits far outweigh any sacrifice you are making. Detach from these sleep-stealing items, and you will quickly divorce your zolpidem.

The common theme here is "too much" or "in excess." Just as overdrugging creates multiple health problems, *overindulging* can also cause considerable harm. Excessive eating and drinking habits not only steal your sleep, they make you fat. Obesity ushers in exceedingly more health issues and then more drugs with more side effects, adding more drugs to keep you on a hamster wheel—which does not adhere to an *undrugged* lifestyle.

Sleep-Sabotaging Food and Drink

- Caffeine
- Alcohol
- Sugar and simple carbohydrates
- Fatty and fried foods
- Spicy foods
- Too much protein
- Low-carb diets
- Too much food, overeating, and hefty portion sizes
- Excitotoxins like MSG, aspartame, and Chinese food
- Food intolerances and allergens

Un-Caffeinate: Don't Consume after Noon

You may love your daily wake-me-up, triple-shot, big kahuna, three-pump mocha latte with caramel and whip, but if you must do it, do it in the morning. Froufrou coffee drinks, supercharged energy drinks, and a Starbucks or Coffee Bean on every corner has driven a caffeine obsession to epidemic proportions, making caffeine the most widely used stimulant in the world. For over 85 percent of American adults, it is the go-to that puts "pep in our step" and replaces an afternoon "slump with a jump."[146] Not surprisingly, caffeine is that sneaky little Grim Reaper of dreams responsible for a majority of nighttime stimulation. In moderate doses, caffeine becomes a nervous system stimulant that causes insomnia by blocking crucial sleep neurotransmitters. It even induces mild physical dependence, explaining the need for daily early-morning coffee-fix freak-outs and solving the mystery behind the long lines of customers eager to spend four bucks for an average-tasting Americano in a disposable cup marked with their name spelled wrong.

Next time a Red Bull craving strikes, be aware caffeine's stimulating effects are not transient or quick to pass and can last an average of eight to ten hours. For healthy individuals, half of caffeine's effects dissipate after five to seven hours. However, for an unlucky few, 12.5 percent of the effects can linger around for greater than twenty hours.[147] If you are more sensitive to caffeine, the stimulating effects may exceed twelve hours, and if you suffer from liver disease, you are especially sensitive to caffeine's effects, since caffeine is processed mainly through the liver.[148]

Follow this simple rule of thumb, "Don't consume after noon." Don't even entertain the thought of an after-dinner espresso. Avoid decaf coffee substitutions as well, as the caffeine content in decaf may still be high enough to disrupt sleep.[149] For most, caffeine consumption after 2:00 p.m. will interfere with your deepest sleep.[150] If you find yourself hitting the wall in the afternoon and in need of pepping, resist the urge to caffeinate by opting for some fresh air and a quick walk instead.

Caffeine is found in many of your favorite products, like chocolate, cocoa, cacao beans, colas and other soft drinks, black tea, green tea (highest in matcha green tea), assorted herbal teas, diet pills, preworkout mixes, energy drinks, analgesics used for migraine headaches, over-the-counter pain relievers and cold medications, and some herbal preparations used for stimulation. Food manufacturers have mastered the skill of sneaking caffeine into foods and are only required to list caffeine as an ingredient if they add it to a food or beverage. Unfortunately, if caffeine naturally occurs in a food product, as it does in coffee, tea, or chocolate, manufacturers do not have to list caffeine as an ingredient.[151] Word to the wise, check all labels and use common sense with top offenders.

Speaking of top offenders, many nutritionists tout quenching late-night sugar cravings with a small square of dark chocolate. The satisfaction may be short-lived as you find yourself struggling to sleep later. *All* chocolate contains caffeine, and the darker the chocolate, the higher the caffeine content. For example, a Hershey's Special-Dark Chocolate bar has 20 mg of caffeine, equivalent to approximately half an ounce of espresso. A 1.55-ounce Hershey's milk chocolate bar contains 12 mg of caffeine, which is roughly equal to three cups of decaf coffee. Chocolate also contains other stimulants, like sugar, tyramine, phenylethylamine, and theobromine, known to increase heart rate and sleeplessness.

Un-caffeinate yourself for insomnia prevention by ridding the following and any similar products:

- Red Bull = 80 mg caffeine = 1 ounce Starbucks espresso

Dr. Lori Arnold, PharmD

- Five-Hour Energy = 200 mg caffeine per 2 ounces = 16 ounces regular coffee
- Mountain Dew = 71 mg caffeine per 12 ounces

Finally, I can't forget to mention that caffeine is a pretty potent diuretic, increasing urinary frequency, which disrupts restful sleep.

Undrugged Tidbit: Avoid the "Cheesy Reaction" Keeping You Awake

Brain hyperarousal, the "cheesy reaction," is caused by the sleep stealer *tyramine*, an amino acid found in aged foods. Avoid fermented, aged, pickled, or spoiled food, including, but not limited to:[152]

- Aged cheeses and hard cheeses
- Aged, dried, fermented, cured, and smoked meats
- Dried and pickled fish
- Eggplant
- Fermented vegetables like kimchi, pickles, or sauerkraut
- Raisins
- Red wine
- Soybeans, soy sauce, tofu, miso, teriyaki sauce
- Tap beer or unpasteurized beer or ale

Alcohol: Stop Your "Wine-ing"

Cease the nightcap and *never* use alcohol as your sleep aid. As I previously stated, it is a misconception that alcohol helps with sleep. Although alcohol is a depressant, it can also be a stimulant. If limited to one *reasonably sized* alcoholic beverage, studies have shown it may help you fall asleep faster. However, you will not get quality sleep.[153]

Numerous adverse effects are often not considered while enjoying a crisp and citrusy glass of pinot grigio or any number of other libations. Alcohol is high in sugar; increases insulin levels; and depletes B vitamins, essential fatty acids, protein, and vital hormonal production of melatonin.[154] Alcohol disrupts REM (rapid eye movement) sleep, the most restorative phase associated with deep dreaming, which causes multiple nighttime awakenings, less restful sleep, and an increase in daytime drowsiness.[155] Frequent sleep interruptions from alcohol should be anticipated from increased snoring and sleep apnea due to relaxing your breathing muscles and from an increase in urgent restroom trips due to alcohol's diuretic effects.[156] If this barrage of side effects isn't reason enough to pass on a pilsner or pinot, alcohol causes dehydration, headaches, night sweats and nightmares, as well as cottonmouth, puffy face, and bloodshot eyes. Ladies again drew the short end of the stick, as research proves alcohol causes women to have more disturbed sleep, more frequent awakenings, and an increase in difficulty falling back to sleep with shorter overall total sleep duration.[157]

American Dietary Guidelines suggest limiting alcohol consumption to one drink a day for women and one to two drinks per day for men. The guidelines also specify consumption is on a single day, not the average consumption over several days. Basically, you can't save up your daily limits for consumption on "Fri-yays!" If you must indulge in libations, do so in moderation and stop drinking at least two to three hours before bed. Some experts even suggest optimal alcohol cutoff time of four to six hours before bed. For every alcoholic beverage consumed, drink an equal number of glasses of water to prevent dehydration and to help metabolize alcohol more efficiently, paying close attention to the total fluid volume consumed before bedtime. To truly adhere to an *undrugged* lifestyle, create a nonalcoholic "mocktail" to avoid alcohol effects altogether. Opt for tart cherry juice with sparkling water and a slice of lime, served in a fancy wine glass. Instead of disrupting sleep, you will be promoting it!

High Fat and High Protein Foods: Lighten Your Load

"Get in my belly!" You and I know that feeling all too well. Dinnertime arrives and you are famished. You close your eyes and get lost in a food fantasy, where you are gorging on a juicy double-decker angus-beef burger loaded with applewood-smoked bacon, grilled Maui sweet onions, and triple cheddar cheese, served on a bed of chili cheese fries, all washed down with a banana milkshake. Obsession and salivation sets in, and you begin to plot the most direct route to Bob's Burger Bonanza. Leave this craving in the fantasy zone;

this meal is entirely inappropriate for nighttime consumption—or any consumption, for that matter. Step back, breathe deeply, count to ten, and think about your plan before acting on it. This food fantasy contains deep-fried trans fats; bloat-stimulating spices and beans; froth-forming dairy; and belch-inducing, saturated fat-laden meat. Basically, this meal is a whole lot of trouble for the average Joe. I won't give bonus points for adding a banana; its benefits cannot rescue you.

Digestion is kicked into high gear after heavy evening eating, throwing your body's equilibrium out of whack. Optimally, you want your digestion to slow by 50 percent at night to allow the body to focus on sleep functions. Under duress from a hefty food load, the body fully activates, directing energy away from sleep.[158] Initially, you may feel satisfied and happy and then satiated and tired, but once you lie down, the pleasant feelings will soon be replaced by discomfort. Large meat portions overstimulate stomach acid production and relax the lower esophageal sphincter, thereby causing acid reflux and heartburn.[159] Fatty foods slow digestion, allowing partially digested foods to linger, thus causing bloating and distention.[160] I guarantee you can anticipate an agonizing, sleepless night of indigestion. Easing your misery with an antacid or "plop, plop, fizz, fizz" is a temporary fix to compensate for bad habits—this is not the *undrugged* way.

Prevent any looming gut disaster by making a wise decision to lighten your load at night. Limit dinner protein portions to three to four ounces of lean meat or seafood. Avoid highly marbled and fatty cuts of meat like steak, roast beef, pork chops, and bacon. Fried foods should be avoided in general, but if you must indulge, do not consume your favorite fried items in the evening. Swap your cooking techniques, opting for baking or boiling foods or eating foods raw, rather than frying. For added variety when cooking, I utilize a slow cooker for many meals, as well as an appliance called a Nuwave oven. The Nuwave is an indoor grill that also works well for crisping French fries or sweet potato chips, without the use of greasy deep-fat fryers. Finally, practice strict portion control. Limit dinner to less than six hundred calories, allowing at least three hours between dinner and bedtime. If you plan on enjoying a bedtime snack, divvy up the six hundred calories between your dinner and snacks.

Spicy Foods: It's Getting Hot in Here

That's a spicy meatball! Although spicy foods are extra flavorful, they quickly can become nighttime, belly-burning bombs, inflaming the digestive tract, aggravating ulcers, and increasing heartburn and acid reflux. In addition to delivering a blazing burn, spices, especially red pepper and black pepper, can also be stimulating. It is postulated that capsaicin, the active ingredient in chili peppers, raises core body temperature, increases wakefulness, and delays falling asleep.[161] To ward off sleep disturbances, restrict your intake of fiery foods.

Sugar and Simple Carbs: Sugar and Spice—Not So Nice

"Me want cookie!" Nightfall may morph you into Cookie Monster, ravenously hunting for sweet treats. Spend some time investigating sugar cravings, as you could be battling possible nutrient deficiencies of chromium, carbon, phosphorus, sulfur, or tryptophan.[162] If you specifically crave chocolate, this could signal a magnesium deficiency.[163] The most effective way to defend yourself from the sugar beast is to create a strong offense—don't keep sugary treats in your house. By making enticing foods less accessible, you remove the temptation that causes you to leap off the deep end.

Insomnia and sleep interruptions often result from blood sugar and hormonal fluctuations. Consuming a bedtime sweet treat causes an initial blood sugar "spike" that gives bursts of energy and stimulation. Though a welcome effect during the day, it is unwanted at night. Your brain thrives on extra glucose, and by feeding it more sugar you rev up your mental capacity, when you should be shutting it down. Newton's law of universal gravitation, also dubbed Newton's second law, tells us "what goes up must come down"; within a couple hours, your blood sugar "dips," inducing reactive sweating, clamminess, and headaches, which ultimately contributes to restlessness and disrupted sleep.

As a whole, Americans eat and drink way too much sugar. According to the United States Department of Agriculture (USDA), in 2009, the average American consumed 130 pounds of sugar (refined sugar, corn sugar, and high fructose corn syrup) yearly, approximately twenty-six 5-pound bags for each and every one of us.[164] You may briefly enjoy the sweet bliss and sugar high, but eventually you will pay an ongoing, enormous price in health consequences, including erratic blood sugar fluctuations, increased insulin production, insulin resistance, increased stress hormones, overgrowth of bad gut bacteria and yeast, decreased immunity, weight gain, diabetes, and heart disease, just to name a few.

Sugar is everywhere. It is estimated that 80 percent of all processed foods contain added sugar.[165] Watch for ingredients ending in "-ose," as this denotes a sugar-containing product—sucrose, dextrose, fructose, glucose, galactose, lactose, high fructose corn syrup (HFCS), and glucose solids. Other clever names for hidden sugar include cane juice, dextrin, maltodextrin, dextran, barley malt, beet sugar, corn syrup, caramel, demerara sugar, buttered syrup, carob syrup, brown sugar, date sugar, malt syrup, molasses, raw sugar, castor sugar, rice syrup, confectioner's sugar, syrup, treacle, D-mannose, honey, diastase, diastatic malt, fruit juice, fruit juice concentrate, golden syrup, turbinado, sorghum syrup, refiner's syrup, ethyl maltol, maple syrup, and yellow sugar.

Avoid all sugars and simple carbs, including bread, pasta, soda, cakes, cookies, pastries, ice cream, candy, and other sugary foods. If you need an alternative sweetener, switch to a sugar substitute that does not cause blood sugar spikes, such as stevia, and safer sugar alcohols, xylitol and non-GMO erythritol. If you desire a nature-made sweetener, consider small quantities of the following acceptable options—organic honey, grade B maple syrup, coconut sugar, dates, and fresh organic fruit.

Satisfy your internal Cookie Monster and avoid middle-of-the-night sugar crashes by replacing nighttime sugar craving with one of the *undrugged* approved bedtime snacks instead. These options will keep your blood sugar and hormone levels stabilized and assure undisrupted sleep.

Low-Carb Diets: Weight Loss Fads Create Sleep Loss

The creation of a carb-phobic craze has been led by Atkins, South Beach, 5:2, Dukan, and ketogenic diets. Consumers enthusiastically join the frenzy because these diets are effective; weight loss is rapid, blood sugar levels stabilize, and loved ones often begin complimenting you on your noticeably shrinking waistline and slimmer face. Cutting out entire food groups long-term is unwise and unsustainable, with many hefty repercussions guaranteed to backfire down the road.

An often-unmentioned significant downside of long-term carb restriction is the eventual disruption of your crucial hormonal symphony, bringing unwanted health issues. Lose the weight; lose the sleep.[166] Severe carb restriction induces ketosis, forcing you to burn stored fat and carbs for energy needs. Ketosis is the key to success with these diets. However, prolonging ketosis for extended periods brings unwanted nausea, fatigue, bad breath, constipation, muscle cramps, headaches, and *insomnia*.[167]

As a replacement for carbs, several ketogenic diets encourage excessive protein and fat consumption, known sleep saboteurs.[168] Meat overloading offsets the body's delicate acid-base balance, causing a highly acidic state that generates increased detrimental prostaglandins that contribute to pain, inflammation, and depression. Consuming excess meat and deficient carbs also causes extreme sugar cravings, as your body desperately struggles to find alternate glucose sources to maintain normal functioning.[169] Your new obsession may soon become "healthified" versions of popular desserts, indulging in protein powder pancakes, mug cakes, muffins, and puddings or becoming addicted to s'mores and cookie dough protein bars and salted caramel protein ice cream. The sugar substitutes found in diet "Frankenfoods" interfere with your ability to judge sweetness, thereby leading to more sugar and carb cravings, binging, and overeating. Nix these sleep-disrupting artificial sweeteners—acesulfame potassium, alitame, aspartame, cyclamate, saccharin, and sucralose.[170]

One final plug for carbs—carb consumption makes you happier.[171] People who eat healthy, complex carbohydrates have a more pleasant disposition and sleep better. On the other hand, people who frequently cycle through diet extremes, restrict carbs, or only load up on protein and fatty foods often have rotten moods, are highly irritable, and suffer from insomnia. To restore normal sleep patterns, practice moderation by reestablishing a healthy relationship with carbs balanced with a reasonable intake of protein and fat.

Excitotoxins: Un-Caffeinated Stimulants

Popular, delicious munching snacks like cheesy poofs and spicy ranch tortilla chips can be addictive and have a way of keeping you coming back for more. You can't stop at just one. What keeps you mindlessly munching, the cheesy crunch, the salty tang, or could it be the other

Dr. Lori Arnold, PharmD

chemical sprinkles on those tasty little morsels? The culprit is most likely excitotoxins, the addictive funfetti chemical sprinkles added to your food. These dangerous chemicals stimulate, excite, damage, and destroy brain cells and are known to cause headaches, rapid heartbeat, and stomach cramping, as well as more serious conditions like depression, paranoia, violent behaviors, sexual development issues, hormonal disorders, and infertility.[172] Add excitotoxins to the list of sleep sabotages, as these potent brain stimulators contribute to restlessness and excitability, counteracting all attempts to relax.[173]

The most common sleep-stealing excitotoxins are MSG (monosodium glutamate) and aspartame. MSG is used to enhance food flavors and stimulate taste buds, keeping you wanting, and purchasing, more Frankenfoods. MSG is found in roughly 80 percent of processed foods and is hidden on labels under the guises of over forty different ingredients, including items attached to these names—autolyzed, glutamate, hydrolyzed, soy protein, nutritional yeast, or natural flavors.[174] MSG is even found in pharmaceutical products like vaccines, including Adenovirus, Influenza (FluMist) Quadrivalent, MMR (MMR-II), MMRV (ProQuad), Rabies (RabAvert), Varicella (Varivax), and Zoster (Shingles - Zostavax).[175] Protein powders may contain a form of MSG, glutamic acid; however, they typically are unadulterated and free of adverse reactions. For glutamic acid to cause reactions, it must be sourced from fermented protein. Finally, MSG effects are amplified by caffeine, so exercise caution when combining processed foods and drinks. For more information on how glutamic acid destroys nerve and brain cells, read the excellent book *Excitotoxins: The Taste That Kills*, by Russell Blaylock.[176]

Aspartame, aspartate, and aspartic acid are found in numerous products, including diet drinks, diet gelatins, sugar-free diet foods, and sugar-free gums and mints.[177] NutraSweet is the most widely recognized aspartame product, and recently manufacturers rebranded aspartame as "AminoSweet," attempting to cleverly hide it under another alias. Similar to MSG, aspartame is linked to neurological side effects such as headaches, dizziness, anxiety, depression, memory loss, confusion, sleep disorders, and seizures.[178] Aspartame is also found in several pharmaceutical products, especially children's medicines.

Besides excitotoxins, many other food additives, like preservatives, artificial colors/flavors/sweeteners, texture enhancers and synthetic antioxidants can disrupt sleep.[179] Don't stress yourself out trying to memorize a long list of food additives, stimulants, and excitotoxins; instead, simply follow the *undrugged* lifestyle by trashing processed junk foods and opting for healthy whole foods.

Undrugged **Tidbit: Avoid "Excitotoxins" for Better Sleep**

Hidden "excitotoxins" can be found in your food products under the following names:

- Anything with *aspartate* in the name, like aspartame, aspartic acid, NutraSweet, AminoSweet
- Anything with *autolyzed* in the name, like autolyzed yeast extract
- Anything with *caseinate* in the name, like calcium caseinate or sodium caseinate
- Anything with *glutamate* in the name, like monosodium glutamate
- Anything with *hydrolyzed* in the name, like hydrolyzed vegetable protein
- Anything with *soy protein* in the name, like soy protein concentrate or soy protein isolate
- Glutamic acid
- Nutritional yeast and yeast extract
- Natural flavor(s)
- Sucralose (Splenda)
- Textured protein

Food Intolerances: Allergic to Sleep

Hidden food sensitivities are sleep wreckers. Sometimes, exposure to common foods, chemical additives, or molds can trigger chronic immune system activation. Unlike a true food allergy, which often manifests as an immediate or life-threatening anaphylactic reaction, food intolerances and sensitivities are a bit sneakier. Usually, the reaction is delayed by a few hours or even a few days and typically presents as gas, bloating, distention, migraines, rash, hives, nasal congestion or runny nose, constipation or diarrhea, and *insomnia*. If you are experiencing any of these symptoms, it is highly probable you are not sleeping well.[180]

If food intolerances are suspect, try a simple elimination of top offending foods like wheat, milk, refined sugar, soy, corn, eggs, peanuts, and shellfish.[181] The most effective method of tackling food intolerances is to work closely with a skilled functional medicine practitioner to help pinpoint the exact food insults.

Conclusion

I want to leave you with just a couple of *Undrugged Sleep* closing remarks. Ultimately, you have the gift of free will, which allows you to take control and determine your future health potential. I have presented you with the option to choose whether you will continue your journey with sleep drugs or whether you will follow an *undrugged* lifestyle. Don't forget, when you know better, you do better; and now you have valuable information to help establish your informed knowledge base. I implore you to seize the opportunity to *do better*.

It is my goal to help instill confidence—to empower you to *trust* in your own judgment before agreeing to any health-related decisions. Going forward, I encourage you to take responsibility for your own body and to resist accepting treatment recommendations at face value; question and investigate all prescription and over-the-counter drugs before ingesting. Asking for a second opinion or inquiring about alternatives when faced with critical health choices is perfectly acceptable, and in many cases, seeking alternative medicine practitioners is warranted. In my professional opinion, any additional drug being added to your regimen constitutes a *critical health choice*. For my personal health and well-being, I am very discerning when I introduce any chemical into my body, and I sincerely hope you become equally as discerning. Pharmaceutical drugs are not "nature made" and, more often than not, are wrought with dozens of unintended consequences.

In most cases, sleep drugs merely create an unstable crutch—merely allowing you to hobble along until eventually you're knocked off your feet. The long-term consequences of pill popping could prove to be much more disastrous than just losing a few nights of sleep over the short-term. Yes, dumping your drug may be painful for a few nights, but once a normal *undrugged* sleep rhythm is established, you will enjoy improvements in overall quality and quantity of your sleep. I suffered as a sleep-deprived insomniac and am now living proof that sleeping pill dependence can be successfully overcome. Though I still suffer from occasional mental stressors that create subpar sleep, I never resort to drug therapy; rather I employ *undrugged* tools to restore productive sleep on a majority of nights. I no longer experience strange or worrisome side effects, and I know with certainty that I am utilizing the safest solutions that are also kind to my body. Be kind to your body. Choose the safest alternative. Join me by becoming a fellow reformed insomniac, living your own *undrugged* lifestyle.

Endnotes

Part I – Are Sleep Drugs Worsening Your Insomnia?

1. Sowder Group LLC, "The Better Sleep Guide," accessed August 4, 2016, https://www.better-sleep-better-life.com/insomnia-medications.html.
2. M. Moloney, T. Konrad, and C. Zimmer, "The Medicalization of Sleeplessness: A Public Health Concern, *American Journal of Public Health* 101, no. 8 (August 2011): 1429–33.
3. Ibid.
4. E. Ford, A. Wheaton, T. Cunningham, W. Giles, D. Chapman, and J. Croft. "Trends in Outpatient Visits for Insomnia, Sleep Apnea, and Prescriptions for Sleep Medications among US Adults: Findings from the National Ambulatory Medical Care Survey 1999–2010, *Sleep* 37, no. 8 (August 2014): 1283–93.
5. Moloney et al., "The Medicalization of Sleeplessness."
6. J. Shepard, D. Buysse, A. Chesson, W. Dement, R. Goldberg, C. Guilleminault, C. Harris, et al., "History of the Development of Sleep Medicine in the United States," *Journal of Clinical Sleep Medicine* 1, No. 1 (January 2005): 61–82.
7. National Institute for Health and Care Excellence, "Guidance on the Use of Zaleplon, Zolpidem and Zopiclone for the Short-Term Management of Insomnia," accessed August 8, 2016, https://www.nice.org.uk/guidance/ta77.
8. Stephanie Saul. "FDA Warns of Sleeping Pills' Strange Effects." *New York Times,* March 17, 2007.
9. Y. Chong, C. Fryer, and Q. Gu, "Prescription Sleep Aid Use among Adults: United States, 2005–2010, *NCHS Data Brief* 127 (August 2013): 1–8.

10   Centers for Disease Control and Prevention (CDC), "Perceived Insufficient Rest or Sleep among Adults – United States, 2008," *Morbidity and Morality Weekly Report* 58 (2009): 1175–79.
11   National Institutes of Health, "National Institutes of Health State of the Science Conference Statement on Manifestations and Management of Chronic Insomnia in Adults, June 13–15, 2005," *Sleep* 28 (2005): 1049–57.
12   American Psychiatric Association, "Sleep-Wake Disorders" in *Diagnostic and Statistical Manual of Mental Disorders, Fifth Edition (DSM-5)*," (Arlington, VA: American Psychiatric Association, 2013).
13   Y. Chong, C. Fryer, and Q. Gu, "Prescription Sleep Aid Use among Adults: United States, 2005–2010, *NCHS Data Brief* 127 (August 2013): 1–8.
14   National Commission on Sleep Disorders Research (U.S.), Department of Health and Human Services, *Wake Up America: A National Sleep Alert* (Washington, DC: The Commission, 1993–1995).
15   R. Knipling and S Wang, *Revised Estimates of the U.S. Drowsy Driver Crash Problem Size Based on General Estimates System Case Reviews, 39th Annual Proceedings* (Chicago: Association for the Advancement of Automotive Medicine, 1995).
16   M. Kuppermann, D. Lubeck, P. Mazoson, D. Patrick, A. Stewart, D. Buesching, and S. Fifer. "Sleep Problems and Their Correlates in a Working Population," *Journal of General Internal Medicine* 10, no. 1 (January 1995): 25–32.
17   Shepard et al., "History of the Development of Sleep Medicine."
18   National Institute for Health and Care Excellence, "Guidance on the Use of Zaleplon, Zolpidem and Zopiclone."
19   K. Adams and E. Breden-Crouse. "Melatonin Agonists in the Management of Sleep Disorders: A Focus on Ramelteon and Tasimelteon," *Mental Health Clinician* 4, no. 2 (March 2014): 59–64.
20   The European Committee for Medicinal Products for Human Use (CHMP), "Ramelteon: Application Withdrawn. Ramelteon in Insomnia: Withdrawal of Marketing Application in Patients' Best Interests," *Prescrire International* 18, no. 101 (June 2009): 114.
21   M. Mieda and T. Sakurai, "Overview of Orexin/Hypocretin System," *Progress in Brain Research* 198 (2012): 5–14.

22 D. McNeil, *Clinical Review NDA 21-774. Zolpidem Tartrate (Ambien CR)* (Silver Spring, MD: Food and Drug Administration, Center for Drug Evaluation and Research, 2005).
23 N. Buscemi, B. Vandermeer, C. Friesen, L. Bialy, M. Tubman, M. Ospina, T. Klassen, and M. Witmans, "The Efficacy and Safety of Drug Treatments for Chronic Insomnia in Adults: A Meta-Analysis of RCTs," *Journal of General Internal Medicine* 22, no. 9 (September 2007): 1335–50.
24 T. Huedo-Medina, I. Kirsch, J. Middlemass, M. Klonizakis, and A. Siriwardena, "Effectiveness of Non-Benzodiazepine Hypnotics in Treatment of Adult Insomnia: Meta-Analysis of Data Submitted to the Food and Drug Administration, *BMJ* 345 (December 2012): e8343.
25 McNeil, *Clinical Review NDA 21-774*.
26 Sanofi Pharmaceuticals, "Ambien (Zolpidem Tartrate) Prescribing Information," accessed July 1, 2016, https://www.products.sanofi.us/ambien/ambien.pdf; Pfizer Pharmaceuticals, "Sonata (Zaleplon) Prescribing Information," accessed July 1, 2016, https://www.pfizer.com/products/product-detail/sonata_civ; Sunovion Pharmaceuticals, "Lunesta (Eszopiclone) Prescribing Information," accessed July 1 2016, https://www.lunesta.com.
27 Buscemi et al., "The Efficacy and Safety of Drug Treatments."
28 Huedo-Medina et al., "Effectiveness of Non-Benzodiazepine Hypnotics."
29 Buscemi et al., "The Efficacy and Safety of Drug Treatments."
30 Huedo-Medina et al., "Effectiveness of Non-Benzodiazepine Hypnotics."
31 Buscemi et al., "The Efficacy and Safety of Drug Treatments."
32 Ibid.
33 P. Nowell, S. Mazumdar, D. Buysse, M. Dew, C. Reynolds, and D. Kupfer, "Benzodiazepines and Zolpidem for Chronic Insomnia: A Meta-Analysis of Treatment Efficacy. *The Journal of the American Medical Association* 278, no. 14 (December 24–31, 1997): 2170–77.
34 A. Qaseem, D. Kansagara, M. Forciea, M. Cooke, and T. Denberg, Clinical Guidelines Committee of the American College of Physicians, "Management of Chronic Insomnia Disorder in Adults: A Clinical Practice Guideline from the American College

of Physicians," *Annals of Internal Medicine* 165, no 2. (July 19, 2016): 125–33.
35 National Institutes of Health, "NIH State-of-the-Science Conference Statement on Manifestations and Management of Chronic Insomnia in Adults," *NIH Consensus and State-of-the Science Statements* 22, no 2 (June 13–15 2005): 1–30.
36 G. Asnis, M. Thomas, and M. Henderson, "Pharmacotherapy Treatment Options for Insomnia: A Primer for Clinicians," *International Journal of Molecular Sciences* 17, no 1 (December 2015): E50.
37 T. Moore, M. Cohen, C. Furberg, and D. Mattison, "ISMP QuarterWatch: Monitoring FDA MedWatch Reports, May 6, 2015," accessed October 6, 2017, https://www.ismp.org/QuarterWatch/pdfs/2014Q2.pdf.
38 J. Buenconsejo, *Statistical Review and Evaluation: Clinical Studies Ambien CR (Zolpidem MR)* (Silver Spring, MD: Food and Drug Administration, Center for Drug Evaluation and Research, 2005).
39 M. Tsai, Y. Huang, and P. Wu, "A Novel Clinical Pattern of Visual Hallucination after Zolpidem Use," *Journal of Toxicology: Clinical Toxicology* 41, no. 6 (2003): 869–72.
40 Sunovion Pharmaceuticals, "Lunesta (Eszopiclone) Prescribing Information"; M. Tsai et al., "A Novel Clinical Pattern."
41 J. Woods, J. Katz, and G. Winger. "Benzodiazepines: Use, Abuse, and Consequences," *Pharmacological Reviews* 44, no. 2 (June 1992): 151–347.
42 D. Kripke, "Chronic Hypnotic Use: Deadly Risks, Doubtful Benefit," *Sleep Medicine Reviews* 4, no. 1 (February 2000): 5–20.
43 Sanofi Pharmaceuticals, "Ambien (Zolpidem Tartrate) Prescribing Information."
44 D. Kripke, S. Ancoli-Israel, M. Klauber, D. Wingard, W. Mason, and D. Mullaney. "Prevalence of Sleep Disordered Breathing in ages 40–64 Years: A Population-Based Survey," *Sleep* 20, no. 1 (January 1997): 65–76; S. Ancoli-Israel, D. Kripke, M. Klauber, W. Mason, R. Fell, and O. Kaplan. "Sleep Disordered Breathing in Community-Dwelling Elderly. *Sleep* 14, no. 6 (December 1991): 486–95.
45 G. Gagliardi, A. Shah, M. Goldstein, S. Denua-Rivera, K. Doghramji, S. Cohen, and A. Dimarino. "Effect of Zolpidem

on the Sleep Arousal Response to Nocturnal Esophageal Acid Exposure," *Clinical Gastroenterology and Hepatology* 7, no. 9 (September 2009): 948–52.
46 F. Joya, D. Kripke, R. Loving, A. Dawson, and L. Kline. "Meta-Analysis of Hypnotics and Infections: Eszopiclone, Ramelteon, Zaleplon, and Zolpidem," *Journal of Clinical Sleep Medicine* 5, no. 4 (August 2009): 377–83; K. Sato and T. Nakashima. "Human Adult Deglutition during Sleep. *Annals of Otology, Rhinology, and Laryngology* 115, no. 5 (May 2006): 334–39.
47 R. Farkas, *Center for Drug Evaluation and Research: Approval Package for: Application Number: 019908Orig1s032s034 021774Orig1s013s015* (Silver Springs, MD: FDA, 2013).
48 Ancoli-Israel et al., "Sleep Disordered Breathing."
49 C. Huang, F. Chou, Y. Huang, C. Yang, Y. Su, S. Juang, P. Chen, P. Chou, C. A. Lee, and C. C. Lee, "The Association between Zolpidem and Infection in Patients with Sleep Disturbances," *Journal of Psychiatric Research* 54, no. 7 (July 2014): 116–20.
50 K. Liao, C. Lin, S. Lai, and W. Chen, "Zolpidem Use Associated with Increased Risk of Pyogenic Liver Abscess," *Medicine* 94, no. 32 (August 2015): e1302.
51 D. Kripke. "Greater Incidence of Depression with Hypnotics Than with Placebo," *BMC Psychiatry* 7 (August 2007): 42.
52 Y. Sun, C. Lin, C. Lu, C. Hsu, and C. Kao. "Association between Zolpidem and Suicide: A Nationwide Population-Based Case-Control Study," *Mayo Clinic Proceedings* 91, no. 3 (March 2016): 308–15.
53 D. Kripke, *FDA Asked to Severely Restrict Use of Most Commonly-Prescribed Sleeping Pills* (La Jolla, CA: Formal Citizen Petition submission to FDA, 2015).
54 D. Kripke D. "Hypnotic Drug Risks of Mortality, Infection, Depression, And Cancer: but Lack of Benefit (version 1; referees: 2 approved)", *F1000Research* 5, no. 918 (2016), doi: 10.12688/f1000research.8729.1.
55 S. Lai, C. Lin, and K. Liao, "Increased Relative Risk of Acute Pancreatitis In Zolpidem Users," *Psychopharmacology* 232, no.12 (June 2015): 2043–48; S. Lai, H. Lai, C. Lin, and K. Liao K, "Zopiclone Use Associated with Increased Risk of Acute Pancreatitis: A Case-Control Study in Taiwan," *International*

Journal of Clinical Practice 69, no. 11 (November 2015): 1275–80.
56 Kripke, "Hypnotic Drug Risks."
57 D. Kripke, R. Langer, and L. Kline, "Hypnotics' Association with Mortality or cancer: A Matched Cohort Study," *BMJ Open* 2 (2012): e000850.
58 C. Kao, L. Sun, J. Liang, S. Chang, F. Sung, and C. Muo, "Relationship of Zolpidem and Cancer Risk: A Taiwanese Population-Based Cohort Study," *Mayo Clinic Procedures* 87, no. 5 (May 2012): 430–36.
59 Kripke, "Hypnotic Drug Risks."
60 American Geriatrics Society 2012 Beers Criteria Update Expert Panel, "American Geriatrics Society Updated Beers Criteria for Potentially Inappropriate Medication Use in Older Adults," *Journal of the American Geriatrics Society* 60, no. 4 (April 2012): 616–31.
61 S. Tom, E. Wickwire, Y. Park, and J. Albrecht, "Non-Benzodiazepine sedative Hypnotics and Risk of Fall-Related Injury," *Sleep* 39, no. 5 (May 1, 2016): 1009–14.
62 S. Berry, Y. Lee, S. Cai, and D. Dore, "Non-Benzodiazepine Sleep Medication Use and Hip Fractures in Nursing Home Residents," *JAMA Internal Medicine* 173, no. 9 (May 2013): 754–61.
63 M. Frisher, N. Gibbons, K. Bashford, S. Chapman, and S. Weich, "Melatonin, Hypnotics and Their Association with Fracture: A Matched Cohort Study," *Age Ageing* 45, no. 6 (November 2016): 801–6; S. Park, J. Ryu, D. Lee, D. Shin, J. Yun, and J. Lee, "Zolpidem Use and Risk of Fractures: A Systematic Review and Meta-Analysis," *Osteoporosis International* 27, no 10 (October 2016): 2935–44.
64 J. Glass, K. Lanctot, N. Herrmann, B. Sproule, and U. Busto, "Sedative Hypnotics in Older People with Insomnia: Meta-Analysis of Risks and Benefits," *BMJ* 331, no. 7526 (November 19, 2005): 1169.
65 L. Hampton, M. Daubresse, H. Chang, G. Alexander, and D. Budnitz. "Emergency Department Visits by Adults for Psychiatric Medication Adverse Events," *JAMA Psychiatry* 71, no 9. (September 2014): 1006–14.
66 Glass et al., "Sedative Hypnotics in Older People."

67 IMS Health, "Top 25 Medicines by Dispensed Prescriptions (U.S.)," accessed October 6, 2017, https://www.imshealth.com/files/web/Corporate/News/Top-Line%20Market%20Data/US_Top_25_Medicines_Dispensed_Prescriptions.pdf.
68 Ibid.
69 Hampton, et al., "Emergency Visits."
70 IMS Health, "Top 25 Medicines."
71 N. Gunja, "In the Zzz Zone: The Effects of Z-drugs on Human Performance and Driving, *The Journal of Medical Toxicology* 9, no. 2 (June 2013): 163–71.
72 IMS Health, "Top 25 Medicines."
73 Gunja, "In the Zzz Zone."
74 T. Inagaki, T. Miyaoka, S. Tsuji, Y. Inami, A. Nishida, and J. Horiguchi, "Adverse Reactions to Zolpidem: Case Reports and a Review of the Literature," *Primary Care Companion to the Journal of Clinical Psychiatry* 12, no. 6 (20106), doi:10.4088/PCC.09r00849bro.
75 C. Elko, J. Burgess, and W. Robertson, "Zolpidem-Associated Hallucinations and Serotonin Reuptake Inhibition: A Possible Interaction," *Journal of Toxicology: Clinical Toxicology* 36, no. 3 (1998): 195–203.
76 L. Toner, B. Tsambiras, G. Catalano, M. Catalano, and D. Cooper, "Central Nervous System Side Effects Associated with Zolpidem Treatment," *Clinical Neuropharmacology* 23, no. 1 (January-February 2000): 54–8.
77 H. Nzwalo, L. Ferreira, R. Peralta, and C. Bentes, "Sleep-Related Eating Disorder Secondary to Zolpidem," *BMJ Case Reports* (February 21, 2013): pii:bcr2012008003.
78 C. Schenck, T. Hurwitz, S. Bundlie, and M. Mahowald, "Sleep-Related Eating Disorders: Polysomnographic Correlates of a Heterogeneous Syndrome Distinct from Daytime Eating Disorders," *Sleep* 14, no 5. (October 1991): 419–31.
79 T. Morgenthaler and M. Silber. "Amnesic Sleep-Related Eating Disorder Associated with Zolpidem," *Sleep Medicine* 3, no. 4 (July 2002): 323–27.
80 Tsai, Huang, and Wu, "A Novel Clinical Pattern."
81 European Medicines Agency Science Medicines Health, Pharmacovigilance Risk Assessment Committee (PRAC), "Assessment Report for Zolpidem-Containing Medicinal

Products. Procedure Number: EMEA/H/A-31/1377," accessed October 6, 2017, https://www.ema.europa.eu/ema/index.jsp?curl=pages/medicines/human/referrals/Zolpidem-containing_medicines/human_referral_prac_000030.jsp&mid=WC0b01ac05805c516f.
82 Kai Falkenberg. "While You Were Sleeping," accessed July 15, 2016, https://www.marieclaire.com/culture/news/a7302/while-you-were-sleeping/; Craig Kapitan, "High-Profile Defendant Gets Jail, Despite Probation Verdict," accessed August 8, 2016, http://www.mysanantonio.com/news/local_news/article/High-profile-defendant-gets-jail-despite-3714370.php.
83 Gunja, "In the Zzz Zone."
84 Ibid.
85 J. Poceta. "Zolpidem Ingestion, Automatisms, and Sleep Driving: A Clinical and Legal Case Series," *Journal of Clinical Sleep Medicine 7*, no. 6 (December 2011): 632–38.
86 U.S. Food and Drug Administration, "FDA Drug Safety Communication: Risk of Next-Morning Impairment after Use of Insomnia Drugs; FDA Requires Lower Recommended Doses for Certain Drugs Containing Zolpidem (Ambien, Ambien CR, Edluar, and Zolpimist)," accessed July 6, 2016, https://www.fda.gov/downloads/Drugs/DrugSafety/UCM335007.pdf.
87 Gunja, "In the Zzz Zone."
88 Inagaki, et al., "Adverse Reactions to Zolpidem."
89 European Medicines Agency Science Medicines Health, PRAC, "Assessment Report for Zolpidem-Containing Medicinal Products."
90 P. Salva and J. Costa, "Clinical Pharmacokinetics and Pharmacodynamics of Zolpidem: Therapeutic Implications," *Clinical Pharmacokinetics 29*, no. 3 (September 1995): 142–53.
91 Toner et al., "Central Nervous System Side Effects."
92 C. Daley, D. McNiel, and R. Binder, "'I Did What?' Zolpidem and the Courts," *The Journal of the American Academy of Psychiatry and the Law 39*, no. 4 (2011): 535–42.
93 C. Paradis, L. Siegel L, and S. Kleinman, "Two Cases of Zolpidem-Associated Homicide," *The Primary Care Companion for CNS Disorders 14*, no. 4 (2012): pii:PCC.12br01363.
94 Natural Medicines Online Database, "Drug-Induced Nutrient Depletions," accessed August 2, 2016, http://www.

naturalmedicines.therapeuticresearch.com; Carol Newall, Linda Anderson, and J. David Phillipson, *Herbal Medicines: A Guide for Health-Care Professionals* (London: The Pharmaceutical Press, 1996); Alan Gaby, Forrest Batz, Rick Chester, and George Constantine, *A–Z Guide to Drug-Herb-Vitamin Interactions: How to Improve Your Health and Avoid Problems When Using Common Medications and Naturals Supplements Together* (New York: Three Rivers Press, 1999); Joseph Boullata and Vincent Armenti, *Handbook of Drug-Nutrient Interactions* (New Jersey: Humana Press Inc., 2004); Earl Mindell and Hester Mundis, *Earl Mindell's New Vitamin Bible: Updated Information on Nutraceuticals, Herbs, Alternative Therapies, Antiaging Supplements, and More* (New York: Grand Central Publishing, 2004); Earl Mindell and Virginia Hopkins, *Prescription Alternatives: Hundreds of Safe, Natural, Prescription-Free, Remedies to Restore and Maintain Your Health* (New York: McGraw Hill Books, 2009); Michael Murray, *Encyclopedia of Nutritional Supplements: The Essential Guide for Improving Your Health Naturally* (New York: Three Rivers Press, 2001); Ross Pelton and James LaValle, *The Nutritional Cost of Prescription Drugs: How to Maintain Good Nutrition While Using Prescription Drugs* (Englewood, CO: Morton Publishing Company, 2000); Nicola Reavley, *The New Encyclopedia of Vitamins, Minerals, Supplements, and Herbs: A Completely Cross-Referenced User's Guide for Optimal Health* (Lanham, MD: M. Evans and Company, 1998); Pamela Wartian-Smith, *What You Must Know about Vitamins, Minerals, Herbs and More: Choosing the Nutrients that are Right for You* (New York: Square One Publishers, 2008).

Part II – From Insomnia to Un-Somnia: *Undrugged* **Solutions to Naturally Promote Sleep**
95   G. Asnis, M. Thomas, and M. Henderson, "Pharmacotherapy Treatment Options for Insomnia: A Primer for Clinicians," *International Journal of Molecular Sciences* 17, no. 1 (December 30, 2015): pii:E50.
96   T. Morgenthaler, M. Kramer, C. Alessi, L. Friedman, B. Boehlecke, T. Brown, J Coleman, et al., "Practice Parameters for the Psychological and Behavioral Treatment of Insomnia:

An Update; An American Academy of Sleep Medicine Report," *Sleep* 29, no. 11 (November 2006): 1415–19.
97 T. Roehrs and T. Roth, "Caffeine: Sleep and Daytime Sleepiness," *Sleep Medicine Reviews* 12, no. 2 (April 2008): 153–62.
98 I. Ebrahim, C. Shapiro, A. Williams, and Fenwick P, "Alcohol and Sleep: Effects on Normal Sleep," *Alcoholism: Clinical and Experimental Research* 37, no. 4 (April 2013): 539–49.
99 C. F. Wang, Y. Sun, and H. Zang, "Music Therapy Improves Sleep Quality in Acute and Chronic Sleep Disorders: A Meta-Analysis of 10 Randomized Studies," *International Journal of Nursing Studies* 51, no. 1 (January 2014): 51–62.
100 P. Berbel, J. Moix J, and s. Quintana, "Music versus Diazepam to Reduce Preoperative Anxiety: A Randomized Controlled Trial," *Revista Española de Anestesiología y Reanimación* 54, no. 6 (June-July 2007): 355–58; L. Yal, "'Brain Music' in the Treatment of Patients with Insomnia," *Neuroscience and Behavioral Physiology* 28, no. 3 (May-June 1998): 330–35; G. De Niet, B. Tiemens, B. Lendemeijer, and G. Hutschemaekers, "Music-Assisted Relaxation to Improve Sleep Quality: Meta-Analysis," *Journal of Advanced Nursing* 65, no. 7 (July 2009): 1356–64.
101 R. Nagendra, N. Maruthai, and B. Kutty, "Meditation and Its Regulatory Role on Sleep," *Frontiers in Neurology* 18, no. 3 (April 2012): 54.
102 Kimberly Pugh, *The Effect of Reiki on Decreasing Episodes of Insomnia and Improving Sleep Patterns* (Boca Raton: Dissertation.com, 2008).
103 S. Petruzzello, D. Landers, B. Hatfield, K. Kubitz, and W. Salazar, "A Meta-Analysis on the Anxiety-Reducing Effects of Acute and Chronic Exercise," *Sports Medicine* 11, no. 3 (March 1991): 143–82.
104 A. King, R. Oman, G. Brassington, D. Bliwise, and W. Haskell, "Moderate-Intensity Exercise and Self-Rated Quality of Sleep in Older Adults: A Randomized Controlled Trial," *JAMA* 277, no. 1 (January 1997): 32–37.
105 C. Streeter, J. Jensen, R. Perlmutter, H. Cabral, H. Tian, D. Terhune, D. Ciraulo, and P. Renshaw, "Yoga Asana Sessions Increase Brain GABA Levels: A Pilot Study," *Journal of Alternative and Complementary Medicine* 13, no. 4 (May 2007): 419–26.

106 C. Streeter, T. Whitfield, L. Owen, T. Rein, S. Karri, A. Yakhkind, and R. Perlmutter, "Effects of Yoga versus Walking on Mood, Anxiety, and Brain GABA Levels: A Randomized Controlled MRS Study," *Journal of Alternative and Complementary Medicine* 16, no. 11 (November 2010): 1145–52.

107 Michelle Goldberg, *The Goddess Pose: The Audacious Life of Indra Devi, the Woman Who Helped Bring Yoga to the West* (New York: Vintage Books, 2016).

108 R. Goncalves and S. Guimaraes-Togeiro, "Drug-Induced Sleepiness and Insomnia: An Update," *Sleep Science* 6, no. 1 (2013): 36–43; Armon Neel, "10 Types of Meds That Can Cause Insomnia," accessed August 7, 2016, http://www.aarp.org/health/drugs-supplements/info-04-2013/medications-that-can-cause-insomnia.html; Harvard Health Publications, Harvard Medical School, "Medications That Can Affect Sleep," accessed August 7, 2016, https://www.health.harvard.edu/newsletter_article/medications-that-can-affect-sleep.; James Tisdale and Douglas Miller, *Drug-Induced Diseases: Prevention, Detection, and Management, Second Edition* (Bethesda, MD: American Society of Health-System Pharmacists, Inc., 2010).

109 P. Bond, "Ten Energy-Boosting Herbs and Supplements," *Natural Foods Merchandiser* XXVII, no. 3 (April 24, 2008): 58–68; A. Eckert, "Mitochondrial Effects of Ginkgo Biloba Extract," *International Psychogeriatrics* 24, suppl 1 (August 2012): S18–20; J. Garrido-Maraver, M. Cordero, M. Oropesa-Avila, A. Vega, M. de la Mata, A. Pavon, and E. Alcocer-Gomez, "Clinical Applications of Coenzyme Q10. *Frontiers in Bioscience* landmark edition, no. 19 (January 1, 2014): 619–33; H. Kim, J. Cho, S. Yoo, J. Lee, J. Han, N. Lee, Y. Ahn, and C. Son, "Anti-Fatigue Effects of *Panax Ginseng* C.A. Meyer: A Randomized, Double-Blind, Placebo-Controlled Trial," *PLOS One* 8, no. 4 (April 2013): e61271.

110 S. Goyal, J. Kaushal, M. Gupta, and S. Verma, "Drugs and Dreams," *Indian Journal of Clinical Practice* 23, no. 10 (March 2013): 624–27.

111 S. Zadeh and K. Begum, Comparison of Nutrient Intake by Sleep Status in Selected Adults in Mysore, India, *Nutrition Research and Practice* 5, no. 3 (June 2011): 230–35.

112 Natural Medicines Online Database, "Drug-Induced Nutrient Depletions," accessed August 2, 2016, http://www.naturalmedicines.therapeuticresearch.com; Carol Newall, Linda Anderson, and J. David Phillipson, *Herbal Medicines: A Guide for Health-Care Professionals* (London: The Pharmaceutical Press, 1996); Alan Gaby, Forrest Batz, Rick Chester, and George Constantine. *A-Z Guide to Drug-Herb-Vitamin Interactions: How to Improve Your Health and Avoid Problems When Using Common Medications and Naturals Supplements Together* (New York: Three Rivers Press, 1999); Joseph Boullata and Vincent Armenti, *Handbook of Drug-Nutrient Interactions* (New Jersey: Humana Press Inc., 2004); Earl Mindell and Hester Mundis, *Earl Mindell's New Vitamin Bible: Updated Information on Nutraceuticals, Herbs, Alternative Therapies, Antiaging Supplements, and More* (New York: Grand Central Publishing, 2004); Mindell, Earl and Virginia Hopkins, *Prescription Alternatives: Hundreds of Safe, Natural, Prescription-Free, Remedies to Restore and Maintain Your Health* (New York: McGraw Hill Books, 2009); Michael Murray, *Encyclopedia of Nutritional Supplements: The Essential Guide for Improving Your Health Naturally* (New York: Three Rivers Press, 2001); Ross Pelton and James LaValle, *The Nutritional Cost of Prescription Drugs: How to Maintain Good Nutrition While Using Prescription Drugs* (Englewood, CO: Morton Publishing Company, 2000); Nicola Reavley, *The New Encyclopedia of Vitamins, Minerals, Supplements, and Herbs: A Completely Cross-Referenced User's Guide for Optimal Health* (Lanham, MD: M. Evans and Company, 1998); Pamela Wartian-Smith; *What You Must Know about Vitamins, Minerals, Herbs and More: Choosing the Nutrients that are Right for You* (New York: Square One Publishers, 2008).

113 E. Ferracioli-Oda, A. Qawasmi, and M. Bloch, "Meta-Analysis: Melatonin for the Treatment of Primary Sleep Disorders," *PLOS One* 8, no. 5 (May 17, 2013) :e63773.

114 B. Abbasi, M. Kimiagar, K. Sadeghniiat, M. Shirazi, M. Hedayati, and B. Rashidkhani B, "The Effect of Magnesium on Primary Insomnia in Elderly: A Double-Blind Placebo-Controlled Clinical Trial," *Journal of Research in Medical Sciences* 17, no. 12 (December 2012): 1161–69.

115 D. Watts, "The Nutritional Relationships of Magnesium," *Journal of Orthomolecular Medicine* 4, no. 4 (1988): 197–201.
116 T. Birdsall, "5-Hydroxytryptophan: A Clinically-Effective Serotonin Precursor," *Alternative Medicine Review* 3, no. 5 (August 1998): 271–80.
117 A. Soulairac and H. Lambinet, "Clinical Studies of the Effect of the Serotonin Precursor, L-5-Hydroxytryptophan on Sleep Disorders," *Schweizerische Rundschau fur Medizin Praxis* 77, no. 34A (August 23, 1988): 19–23.
118 Eric Braverman, *The Healing Nutrients Within* (Laguna Beach: Basic Health Publications, 2003); Thorne Research, "Gamma-Aminobutyric Acid (GABA)," *Alternative Medicine Review* 12, no. 3 (September 2007): 274–79.
119 W. Shell, D. Bullias, E. Charuvastra, L. May, and Silver D, "A randomized, Placebo-Controlled Trial of an Amino Acid Preparation on Timing and Quality of Sleep," *American Journal of Therapeutics* 17, no. 2 (March-April 2010): 133–39.
120 M. McCarty, "High-Dose Pyridoxine as an 'Anti-Stress' Strategy," *Medical Hypotheses* 54, no. 5 (May 2000): 803–7.
121 Trudy Scott, *The Anti-Anxiety Food Solution: How the Foods You Eat Can Help You Calm Your Anxious Mind, Improve Your Mood and End Cravings* (Oakland: New Harbinger Publications, Inc., 2011).
122 S. Bent, A. Padula, D. Moore, M. Patterson, and W. Mehling, "Valerian For Sleep: A Systematic Review and Meta-Analysis," *American Journal of Medicine* 119, no. 12 (December 2006): 1005–12.
123 M. Fernandez-San-Martin, R. Masa-Font, L. Palacios-Soler, P. Sancho-Gomez, C. Calbo-Caldentey, and G. Flores-Mateo G, "Effectiveness of Valerian on Insomnia: A Meta-Analysis of Randomized Placebo-Controlled Trials," *Sleep Medicine* 11, no. 6 (June 2010): 505–11.
124 E. Abourashed, U. Koetter, and A. Brattstrom, "In Vitro Binding Experiments with Valerian, Hops and Their Fixed Combination Extract (Ze91019) to Selected Central Nervous System Receptors," *Phytomedicine* 11, no. 7–8 (November 2004): 633–38; A. Brattstrom, "Scientific Evidence for a Fixed Extract Combination (Ze91019) from Valerian and Hops Traditionally Used as a Sleep-Inducing Aid," *Weiner Medizinsche Wochenschrift* 157,

no. 13–14 (2007: 367–70; S. Salter and S. Brownie, "Treating Primary Insomnia – The Efficacy of Valerian and Hops," *Australian Family Physician* 39, no. 6 (June 2010): 433–37.
125 P. Chan, T. Huang, Y. Chen, W. Huang, and Y. Liu Y, "Randomized, Double-Blind, Placebo-Controlled Study of the Safety and Efficacy of Vitamin B Complex in the Treatment of Nocturnal Leg Cramps in Elderly Patients with Hypertension," *Journal of Clinic Pharmacology* 38, no. 12 (December 1998): 1151–54; C. Earley, R. Allen, J. Beard, and J. Connor J, "Insight into the Pathophysiology of Restless Leg Syndrome," *Journal of Neuroscience Research* 62, no. 5 (December 1, 2000): 623–28.
126 C. Earley, J. Connor, J. Beard, E. Malecki, D. Epstein, and Allen R, "Abnormalities in CSF Concentrations of Ferritin and Transferrin in Restless Leg Syndrome," *Neurology* 54, no. 8 (April 2000): 1698–700.
127 K. Shinomiya, T. Inoue, Y. Utsu, S. Tokunaga, T. Masuoka, A. Ohmori, and C. Kamei C, "Hypnotic Activities of Chamomile and Passiflora Extracts in Sleep-Disturbed Rats," *Biological and Pharmaceutical Bulletin* 28, no. 5 (May 2005): 808–10; H. Viola, C. Wasowski, M. Levi de Stein, C. Wolfman, R. Silveira, F. Dajas, J. Medina, and A. Paladini. "Apigenin, a Component of *Matricaria recutita* Flowers, Is a Central Benzodiazepine Receptors-Ligand with Anxiolytic Effects," *Planta Medica* 61, no. 3 (June 1995): 213–16.
128 J. Sarris Sarris, A. Panossian, I. Schweitzer, C. Stough, and A. Scholey, "Herbal Medicine for Depression, Anxiety and Insomnia: A Review of Psychopharmacology and Clinical Evidence," *European Neuropsychopharmacology* 21, no. 12 (December 2011): 841–60; R. Avallone, P. Zanoli, L. Corsi, G. Cannazza, and M. Baraldi, "Benzodiazepine Compounds and GABA in Flower Heads of *matricaria chamomilla*," *Phytotherapy Research* 10 (1996): S177–79; J. Srivastava, E. Shankar, and S. Gupta, "Chamomile: A Herbal Medicine of the Past with Bright Future," *Molecular Medicine Reports* 3, no. 6 (November 1, 2010): 895–901.
129 S. Akhondzadeh, H. Naghavi, M. Vazirian, A. Shayeganpour, H. Rashidi, and M. Khani, "Passionflower in the Treatment of Generalized Anxiety: A Pilot Double-Blind Randomized

Controlled Trial with Oxazepam," *Journal of Clinical Pharmacy and Therapeutics* 25, no. 5 (October 2001): 363–67.
130 H. S. Jang, J. Jung, I. S. Jang, K. H. Jang, S. Kim, J. Ha, K. Suk, and M. Lee, "L-Theanine Partially Counteracts Caffeine-Induced Sleep Disturbances in Rats," *Pharmacology Biochemistry and Behavior* 101, no. 2 (April 2012): 217–21; K. Kimura, M. Ozeki, L. Juneja, and H. Ohira, "L-Theanine Reduces Psychological and Physiological Stress Responses," *Biological Psychology* 74, no. 1 (January 2007): 39–45.
131 M. Kritsidima, T. Newton, and K. Asimakopoulou, "The Effects of Lavender Scent on Dental Patient Anxiety Levels: A Cluster Randomized-Controlled Trial," *Community Dentistry and Oral Epidemiology* 38, no. 1 (February 2010): 83–87.
132 M. Hardy, M. Kirk-Smith, and D. Stretch, "Replacement of Chronic Drug Treatment of Insomnia in Psychogeriatric Patients by Ambient Odour," *Lancet* 346, no. 8976 (September 9, 1995): 701; G. Lewith, A. Godfrey, and P. Prescott, "A Single-Blinded, Randomized Pilot Study Evaluating the Aroma of *Lavandula augustifolia* as a Treatment for Mild Insomnia," *Journal of Alternative and Complementary Medicine* 11, no. 4 (August 2005): 631–37; C. Graham, "Complementary Therapies: In the Scent of a Good Night's Sleep," *Nursing Standard* 9, no. 21 (1995); M. Ju, S. Lee, I. Bae, M. Hur, K. Seong, and M. Lee, "Effects of Aroma Massage on Home Blood Pressure, Ambulatory Blood Pressure, and Sleep Quality in Middle-Aged Women with Hypertension," *Evidence-Based Complementary and Alternative Medicine* (2013): 403251.
133 M. Cho, E. Min, M. Hur, and M. Lee, "Effects of Aromatherapy on the Anxiety, Vital Signs, and Sleep Quality of Percutaneous Coronary Intervention Patients in Intensive Care Units," *Evidence-Based Complementary and Alternative Medicine* (2013): 381381.
134 T. Komori, T. Matsumoto, M. Yamamoto, E. Motomura, T. Shiroyama, and Y. Okazaki, "Application of Fragrance in Discontinuing the Long-Term Use of Hypnotic Benzodiazepines," *International Journal of Aromatherapy* 16, no. 1 (2006): 3–7; S. Bais, N. Gill, N, Rana, and S. Shandil, "A Phytopharmacological Review on a Medicinal Plant: *Juniperus communis*," *International Scholarly Research Notices* (November 11, 2014): 634723; G.

Cannard, "The Effect of Aromatherapy in Promoting Relaxation and Stress Reduction in a General Hospital," *Complementary Therapies in Nursing and Midwifery* 2, no. 2 (April 1996): 38–40.

135 Ju et al., "Effects of Aroma Massage"; Cannard, "The effect of Aromatherapy"; K. Tastan, M. Isik, R. Sebnem-Yakisan, U. Avsar, and T. Set, "Complementary-Alternative Methods and Cognitive Behavioral Therapies in the Management of Sleep Disorders. *Eurasian Journal of Family Medicine* 2, no. 3 (2013): 101–6; H. N. Jung and H. J. Choi, "Effects of *Organum majorana* Essential Oil Aroma on the Electroencephalograms of Female Young Adults with Sleep Disorders," *Journal of Life Science* 22, no. 8 (2012): 1077–1084.

136 Cho et al., "Aromatherapy in Intensive Care Units"; Tastan et al., "Complementary-Alternative Methods, Cognitive Behavioral Therapies in Sleep Disorders."

137 Ito, Y. Akahoshi, M. Ito, and S. Kaneko, "Sedative Effects of Inhaled Essential Oil Components of Traditional Fragrance *Pogostemon cablin* Leaves and Their Structure-Activity Relationships," *Journal of Traditional Complementary Medicine* 6, no. 2 (February 23, 2015): 140–45; K. Ito and M. Ito, "Sedative Effects of Vapor Inhalation of the Essential Oil of *Microtoena patchouli* and Its Related Compounds," *Journal of Natural Medicine* 65, no. 2 (April 2011): 336–43.

138 A. Ohmori, K. Shinomiya, Y. Utsu, S. Tokunaga, Y. Hasegawa, and C. Kamei, "Effect of Santalol on the Sleep-Wake Cycle in Sleep-Disturbed Rats," *Nihon Shinkei Seishin Yakurigaku Zasshi* 27, no. 4 (August 2007): 167–71; G. Kyle, "Evaluating the Effectiveness of Aromatherapy in Reducing Levels of Anxiety in Palliative Care Patients: Results of a Pilot Study," *Complementary Therapies in Clinical Practice* 12, no. 2 (May 2006): 148–55; B. Misra and S. Dey, "Biological Activities of East Indian Sandalwood Tree, *Santalum album*," *PeerJ Preprints* (November 12, 2013): doi:10.7287/peerj.preprints.96v1; N. Solanki, C. Chauhan, B. Vyas, and D. Marothia, "Santalum Album Linn: A Review," *International Journal of PharmTech Research* 7, no. 4 (2014 –2015;7): 629–40.

139 J. Ilmberger, E. Heuberger, C. Mahrhofer, H. Dessovic, D. Kowarik, and G. Buchbauer, "The Influence of Essential Oils

on Human Attention. I: Alertness," *Chemical Senses* 26, no. 3 (March 2001): 239–45.
140 S. Halder and K. Khaled, "An Extensive Review on the Relationship between Food and Mood," *International Journal of Scientific Research* 5, no. 5 (May 2016): 1750–55.
141 G. Howatson, P. Bell, J. Tallent, B. Middleton, M. McHugh, and J. Ellis, "Effect of Tart Cherry Juice (*Prunus cerasus*) on Melatonin Levels and Enhanced Sleep Quality," *European Journal of Nutrition* 51, no. 8 (December 2012): 909–16.
142 W. Pigeon, M. Carr, C. Gorman, and M. Perlis, "Effects of a Tart Cherry Juice Beverage on the Sleep of Older Adults with Insomnia: A Pilot Study," *Journal of Medicinal Food* 13, no. 3 (June 2010): 579–83.
143 J. Porter and J. Horne, "Bed-Time Food Supplements and Sleep: Effects of Different Carbohydrate Levels," *Electroencephalography and Clinical Nuerophysiology* 51, no. 4 (April 1981): 426–33.
144 C. Hudson, S. Hudson, T. Hecht, and J. MacKenzie, "Protein Source Tryptophan versus Pharmaceutical Grade Tryptophan as an Efficacious Treatment for Chronic Insomnia," *Nutritional Neuroscience* 8, no. 2 (April 2005): 121–27.
145 David Winston, *Adaptogens: Herbs for Strength, Stamina, and Stress Relief* (Rochester: Healing Arts Press, 2007); Michael Tierra, *Planetary Herbology* (Twin Lakes: Lotus Press, 1988).
146 T. McLellan, J. Caldwell, and H. Lieberman, "A Review of Caffeine's Effects on Cognitive, Physical and Occupational Performance," *Neuroscience and Biobehavioral Reviews* 71 (December 2016): 294–312.
147 B. Statland and T. Demas, "Serum Caffeine Half-Lives. Healthy Subjects vs. Patients Having Alcoholic Hepatic Disease," *American Journal of Clinical Pathology* 73, no. 3 (March 1980): 390–93.
148 I. Clark and H. Landolt, "Coffee, Caffeine, and Sleep: A Systematic Review of Epidemiological Studies and Randomized Controlled Trials," *Sleep Medicine Reviews* 31 (February 2017): 70–78.
149 R. McCusker, B. Goldberger, and E. Cone, "Caffeine Content of Specialty Coffees," *Journal of Analytical Toxicology* 27, no. 7 (October 2003): 520–22.

150 L. Shilo, H. Sabbah, R. Hadari, S. Kovatz, U. Weinberg, S. Dolev, Y. Dagan, and L. Shenkman, "The Effects of Coffee Consumption on Sleep and Melatonin Secretion," *Sleep Medicine* 3, no. 3 (May 2002): 271–73.
151 L. Rosenfeld, J. Mihalov, S. Carlson, and A. Mattia, "Regulatory Status of Caffeine in the United States," *Nutrition Reviews* 72, suppl. 1 (October 2014): 23–33.
152 B. McCabe-Sellers, C. Staggs, and M. Bogle, "Tyramine in Foods and Monoamine Oxidase Inhibitor Drugs: A Crossroad Where Medicine, Nutrition, Pharmacy, and Food Industry Converge," *Journal of Food Composition and Analysis* 19 (2006): S58–65.
153 Ebrahim et al., "Alcohol and Sleep"; M. Mahesh, R. Sharma, and P. Sahota, "Alcohol Disrupts Sleep Homeostasis," *Alcohol* 49, no. 4 (June 2015): 299–310.
154 T. Roehrs and T. Roth, "Sleep, Sleepiness, and Alcohol Use," *Alcohol Research & Health* 25, no. 2 (January 2001): 101–9.
155 H. Landolt and A. Borbely, "Alcohol and Sleep Disorders," *Therapeutische Umschau* 57, no. 4 (April 2000): 241–45.
156 M. Scanlan, T. Roebuck, P. Little, J. Redman, and M. Naughton, "Effect of Moderate Alcohol upon Obstructive Sleep Apnoea," *European Respiration Journal* 16, no. 5 (November 2000): 909–13.
157 H. Williams, A. MacLean, and J. Cairns, "Dose-Response Effects of Ethanol in the Sleep of Young Women," *Journal of Studies on Alcohol and Drugs* 44, no. 3 (May 1983): 515–23.
158 M. St-Onge, A. Mikic, and C. Pietrolungo, "Effects of Diet on Sleep Quality," *Advances in Nutrition* 7, no. 5 (September 2016): 938–49.
159 J. Lacey, C. Hawkins, and A. Crisp, "Effects of Dietary Protein on Sleep EEG in Normal Subjects," *Advances in Bioscience* 21 (July 24-25, 1978): 245–47.
160 M. Grandner, D. Kripke, N. Naidoo, and R. Langer, "Relationships among Dietary Nutrients and Subjective Sleep, Objective Sleep, and Napping in Women," *Sleep Medicine* 11, no. 2 (February 2010): 180–84.
161 S. Edwards, I. Montgomery, E. Colquhoun, J. Jordan, and M. Clark, "Spicy Meal Disturbs Sleep: An Effect of Thermoregulation?" *International Journal of Psychophysiology* 13, no. 2 (September 1992): 97–100.

162 K. Bruinsma and D. Taren, "Chocolate: Food or Drug?" *Journal of the American Dietetic Association* 99, no. 10 (October 1999): 1249–56.
163 J. Rodin, J. Mancuso, J. Granger, and E. Nelbach, "Food Cravings in Relation to Body Mass Index, Restraint and Estradiol Levels: A Repeated Measures Study in Healthy Women," *Appetite* 17, no. 3 (December 1991): 177–85.
164 G. Anderson, "Sugars and Health: a Review," *Nutrition Research* 17, no. 9 (September 1997): 1485–98; R. Johnson, L. Appel, M. Brands, B. Howard, M. Lefevre, R. Lustig, F. Sacks, et al., "Dietary Sugars Intake and Cardiovascular Health: A Scientific Statement from the American Heart Association," *Circulation* 120, no. 11 (September 15, 2009): 1011–20; USDA, "Health and Nutrition: Per Capita Consumption of Major Food Commodities," in Statistical Abstract of the United States, 2012, accessed October 6, 2017, https://www.census.gov/library/publications/2011/compendia/statab/131ed/health-nutrition.html.
165 R. Ervin and C. Ogden, "Consumption of Added Sugars among U.S. Adults, 2005-2010." *NCHS Data Brief* 122 (May 2013): 1–8.
166 A. Afaghi, H. O'Connor, and C. Chow, "Acute Effects of the Very Low Carbohydrate Diet on Sleep Indices," *Nutritional Neuroscience* 11, no. 4 (August 2008): 146–54.
167 G. Hajak, A. Rodenbeck, J. Staedt, B. Bandelow, G. Huether, and E. Ruther, "Nocturnal Plasma Melatonin Levels in Patients Suffering from Chronic Primary Insomnia, *Journal of Pineal Research* 19, no. 3 (October 1995): 116–22.
168 G. Lindseth, P. Lindseth, and M. Thompson M, "Nutritional Effects on Sleep," *Western Journal of Nursing Research* 35, no. 4 (April 2013): 497–513.
169 K. Gendall, P. Joyce, and R. Abbott, "The Effects of Meal Composition on Subsequent Craving and Binge Eating," *Addictive Behaviors* 24, no. 3 (May–June 1999): 305–15; K. Stein, "High-Protein, Low-Carbohydrate Diets: Do They Work? *Journal of the American Dietetic Association* 100, no. 7 (July 2000): 760–61.
170 Q. Yang, "Gain Weight by 'Going Diet?' Artificial Sweeteners and the Neurobiology of Sugar Cravings," *Yale Journal of Biology of Medicine* 83, no. 2 (June 2010): 101–8.

171 D. Benton and R. Donohoe, "The Effects of Nutrients on Mood," *Public Health Nutrition* 2, no. 3A (September 1999): 403–9.
172 Russell Blaylock, *Excitotoxins: The Taste That Kills* (Santa Fe, New Mexico: Health Press, 1997); G. Settipane, "The Restaurant Syndromes," *New England and Regional Allergy Proceedings* 8, no. 1 (January–February 1987): 39–46.
173 T. Vaughan, "The Role of Food in the Pathogenesis of Migraine Headache," *Clinical Reviews in Allergy* 12, no. 2 (Summer 1994): 167–80.
174 Truth in Labeling Campaign, "Names of ingredients That Contain Processed Free Glutamic Acid (MSG)," accessed October 1, 2016, www.truthinlabeling.org/hiddensources_printable.pdf.
175 U.S. Centers for Disease Control and Prevention (CDC), "Vaccine Excipient and Media Summary: Ingredients of Vaccines – Fact Sheet," accessed October 6, 2017, https://www.cdc.gov/vaccines/vac-gen/additives.htm.
176 Blaylock, *Excitotoxins*.
177 H. Roberts, "Aspartame (NutraSweet) Addiction," *Townsend Letter for Doctors and Patients* (2000): 52 –57.
178 H. Roberts, "Reactions Attributed to Aspartame-Containing Products: 551 Cases," *Journal of Applied Nutrition* 40 (1988): 85–94; M. Bradstock, M. Serdula, J. Marks, R. Barnard, N. Crane, P. Remington, and F. Trowbridge, "Evaluation of Reactions to Food Additives: The Aspartame Experience," *American Journal of Clinical Nutrition* 43, no. 3 (March 1986): 464–69.
179 B. Wuthrich, "Adverse Reactions to Food Additives," *Annals of Allergy* 71 (1993): 379–84; H. Steinman, "Clinical Approach to Adverse Reactions to Food Additives," *Continuing Medical Education* 23, no. 9 (2005): 439.
180 Rudy Rivera and Roger Davis Deutsch, *Your Hidden Food Allergies Are Making You Fat: How to Lose Weight and Gain Years of Vitality* (New York: Three Rivers Press, 2002).
181 C. Ortolani, C. Bruijnzeel-Koomen, U. Bengtsson, C. Bindslev-Jensen, B. Bjorksten B, A. Host, and M. Ispano, et al., "Controversial Aspects of Adverse Reactions to Food," *Allergy* 54 (1999): 27–45.

Index

1-9

5-HTP (5-hydroxytryptophan) 87, 88, 91, 131
528 Hz Solfeggio 69, 70
(ACP) Chronic Insomnia Guidelines 25

A

Acid reflux xi, 10, 31, 32, 55, 64, 110, 111
Affirmations 61, 69, 70, 75
Alcohol 13, 14, 19, 28, 30, 33, 44, 45, 47, 65, 80, 84, 86, 88, 89, 90, 100, 106, 108, 109, 112, 128, 136
Ambient light 70
Ambien (zolpidem) xi, xv, 3, 4, 5, 12, 14, 23, 24, 26, 31, 32, 33, 34, 35, 36, 37, 38, 39, 40, 41, 42, 43, 44, 45, 47, 48, 54, 55, 56, 57, 59, 60, 61, 82, 91, 105, 119, 120, 121, 122, 123, 124, 125, 126
Apigenin 92, 132
Aromatherapy xvi, 83, 84, 93, 94, 95, 98, 133, 134
Aspartame 106, 113, 114, 115, 138
Asthma x, 10, 31, 72, 80

B

Belsomra (suvorexant) 12, 16

C

Caffeine 9, 14, 22, 65, 80, 90, 106, 107, 108, 114, 128, 133, 135, 136
Cancer 34, 35, 85, 123, 124
Chamomile 6, 92, 95, 96, 98, 132
Chocolate 40, 64, 107, 111, 137
Cognitive Behavioral Therapy (CBT) 57
Complex carbs 104
Complex sleep-related behaviors 30
  Sleep driving xv, 30, 38, 42, 43, 126
  Sleep eating xv, 30, 38, 40, 41
  Sleep sex xv, 30, 38, 48

D

Death 13, 31, 34, 35, 48, 56, 81
Deep belly breathing 74
Dependence 14, 17, 26, 27, 31, 59, 61, 106, 118
Depression xi, 10, 20, 31, 32, 33, 48, 49, 50, 54, 82, 85, 86, 87, 89, 90, 97, 113, 114, 123, 132

Diets 55, 106, 107, 112, 113, 114, 136, 137
   5:2 112
   Atkins 112
   Dukan 112
   Ketogenic 112, 113
   South Beach 112
Dopamine 76, 88
Drug-induced disease xv, 32, 78, 129

E

Edluar (zolpidem) xi, xv, 3, 4, 5, 12, 14, 23, 24, 26, 31, 32, 33, 34, 35, 36, 37, 38, 39, 40, 41, 42, 43, 44, 45, 47, 48, 54, 55, 56, 57, 59, 60, 61, 82, 91, 105, 119, 120, 121, 122, 123, 124, 125, 126
Essential oils 73, 75, 93, 94, 95, 97, 98, 134
Eszopiclone (Lunesta) 5, 12, 23, 24, 28, 31, 33, 121, 122, 123
Excitotoxins 106, 113, 114, 115, 138
Exercise 7, 8, 54, 63, 76, 94, 97, 104, 114, 128

F

Food intolerance 55, 106, 115, 116

G

GABA Calm 91
GABA (gamma-aminobutyric acid) 14, 31, 49, 76, 77, 88, 90, 91, 92, 128, 129, 131, 132
GERD 10, 32
Green tea 65, 80, 92, 107

H

Hallucinations 27, 30, 33, 38, 40, 45, 50, 122, 125
Herbal teas 65, 73, 92, 107
Herbs xiv, xvi, 6, 13, 61, 78, 80, 81, 83, 85, 90, 102, 127, 129, 130, 135
Hippocrates 83, 100
Hz Solfeggio 69

I

Insomnia xi, xv, xvi, 1, 3, 4, 5, 6, 7, 8, 9, 10, 11, 12, 13, 15, 18, 19, 20, 22, 23, 24, 25, 27, 31, 33, 49, 50, 51, 53, 54, 56, 57, 59, 61, 63, 66, 69, 74, 75, 78, 83, 84, 86, 88, 90, 91, 92, 96, 97, 98, 100, 105, 106, 107, 111, 113, 116, 119, 120, 121, 122, 124, 126, 127, 128, 129, 130, 131, 132, 133, 135, 137
   Anxiety-induced 91
   Caffeine-induced 90, 133
   Tired-and-wired 91
Insomnitol 91
Intermezzo (zolpidem) xi, xv, 3, 4, 5, 12, 14, 23, 24, 26, 31, 32, 33, 34, 35, 36, 37, 38, 39, 40, 41, 42, 43, 44, 45, 47, 48, 54, 55, 56, 57, 59, 60, 61, 82, 91, 105, 119, 120, 121, 122, 123, 124, 125, 126

J

Jasmine oil 98
Juniper Berry oil 95, 98

K

Ketosis 113

L

Lavender oil 94, 98
L-theanine 91, 92, 133
Lunesta (eszopiclone) 5, 12, 23, 24, 28, 31, 33, 121, 122, 123

M

Magnesium 84, 86, 87, 88, 91, 94, 101, 103, 111, 130, 131
Meditation 6, 7, 69, 73, 74, 75, 76, 94, 96, 128
Melatonin 6, 10, 12, 15, 67, 84, 85, 86, 87, 88, 91, 101, 102, 103, 104, 108, 120, 124, 130, 135, 136, 137
Mindful eating 64
MSG (monosodium glutamate) 106, 114, 115, 138
Music 14, 58, 69, 73, 94, 128

N

Nightmares x, 37, 38, 81, 85, 95, 101, 109
Norepinephrine 76
Nutraceutical xvi, 6, 15, 41, 55, 57, 84, 127, 130
NutraSweet 114, 115, 138
Nutrient depletions xiv, xv, 49, 126, 130

O

Orexin 12, 16, 120

P

Pancreatitis 33, 123

Parasomnias 37, 38, 39, 40, 41, 42, 43
Passionflower 92, 132
Patchouli oil 96
PharmaGABA 91
Placebo comparator 21
Placebo response 21, 22
Prayer 6, 7, 29, 69, 75, 94, 96
Protein 40, 45, 64, 65, 89, 103, 104, 106, 108, 109, 110, 113, 114, 115, 135, 136, 137
Publication bias 21
Pyridoxine (vitamin B6) 84, 85, 86, 87, 88, 89, 91, 101, 103, 131

R

Ramelteon (Rozerem) 12, 15, 16, 120, 123
Rebound insomnia 25, 27, 31, 57, 59
Reiki 73, 75, 96, 128
Restless Leg Syndrome (RLS) 5, 9, 91, 132
Roman Chamomile oil 96, 98
Rozerem (ramelteon) 12, 15, 16, 120, 123

S

Sandalwood oil 97, 98
Schisandra berries 105
Serotonin 67, 76, 87, 88, 101, 104, 125, 131
Side effects x, xi, xv, 13, 14, 16, 19, 23, 24, 28, 29, 30, 31, 35, 38, 39, 41, 45, 55, 56, 57, 60, 78, 81, 84, 85, 86, 87, 89, 90, 93, 105, 109, 114, 118, 125, 126
Simple carbs 111, 112

Sleep x, xi, xv, xvi, 1, 3, 4, 5, 6, 7, 8, 9, 10, 11, 12, 13, 14, 15, 16, 17, 18, 19, 20, 22, 23, 24, 25, 26, 27, 28, 29, 30, 31, 33, 34, 37, 38, 39, 40, 41, 42, 43, 44, 45, 46, 48, 51, 53, 54, 55, 56, 57, 60, 61, 62, 63, 64, 65, 66, 67, 68, 69, 70, 71, 72, 73, 75, 76, 77, 78, 79, 80, 81, 82, 83, 84, 85, 86, 87, 88, 90, 91, 92, 93, 94, 95, 98, 100, 101, 102, 103, 104, 105, 106, 107, 108, 109, 110, 111, 112, 113, 114, 115, 117, 118, 119, 120, 122, 123, 124, 125, 126, 127, 128, 129, 130, 131, 132, 133, 134, 135, 136, 137
  Apnea 9, 20, 30, 31, 109, 119
  Efficiency 20, 24
  Hygiene 41, 61, 64, 83, 98
  Latency 20, 23
  Maintenance 20, 25, 57
  Promoting foods 61
  Sabotaging foods 100, 105, 106
Sleepwalking xv, 30, 38, 41, 42, 47
Snoring 98, 99, 109
Solfeggio 69, 73, 94
Somnambulism 41
Sonata (zaleplon) 12, 23, 24, 119, 120, 121, 123
Spicy foods 106, 111
Stress x, 10, 13, 20, 42, 57, 64, 68, 69, 70, 72, 73, 74, 75, 76, 77, 87, 88, 89, 92, 94, 95, 97, 98, 102, 112, 114, 131, 133, 134, 135
Sugar 9, 20, 21, 22, 24, 26, 65, 88, 100, 103, 104, 106, 107, 108, 111, 112, 113, 114, 116, 137
Suicide 13, 14, 33, 123
Supplements xi, xiv, xvi, 6, 15, 61, 78, 80, 81, 83, 84, 85, 102, 104, 105, 127, 129, 130, 135
Suvorexant (Belsomra) 12, 16
Sweet Marjoram oil 95, 98

T

Tart cherry juice 102, 109, 135
Tolerance 13, 26, 27, 31, 35, 63, 87
Toxic mold poisoning 75
Tyramine 107, 108, 136

V

Valerian root 90
Vitamin B6 (pyridoxine) 84, 85, 86, 87, 88, 89, 91, 101, 103, 131

W

Wholetones 69, 70
Withdrawal 27, 31, 57, 120

Y

Yoga 70, 76, 77, 96, 128, 129

Z

Zaleplon (Sonata) 12, 23, 24, 119, 120, 121, 123
Z-drugs xv, 3, 4, 5, 12, 14, 15, 17, 18, 19, 20, 21, 22, 23, 24, 25, 26, 27, 28, 29, 30, 31, 32, 33, 34, 35, 38, 42, 44, 45, 46, 49, 56, 57, 60, 76, 125
Z-hypnotics 12, 14

Zolpidem (Ambien) xi, xv, 3, 4,
    5, 12, 14, 23, 24, 26, 31,
    32, 33, 34, 35, 36, 37, 38,
    39, 40, 41, 42, 43, 44, 45,
    47, 48, 54, 55, 56, 57, 59,
    60, 61, 82, 91, 105, 119,
    120, 121, 122, 123, 124,
    125, 126
Zolpidem defense xv, 47, 48
Zolpidem zombies xv, 37, 38, 41
Zolpimist (zolpidem) xi, xv, 3, 4,
    5, 12, 14, 23, 24, 26, 31,
    32, 33, 34, 35, 36, 37, 38,
    39, 40, 41, 42, 43, 44, 45,
    47, 48, 54, 55, 56, 57, 59,
    60, 61, 82, 91, 105, 119,
    120, 121, 122, 123, 124,
    125, 126